What Color Is Your
Swimming Pool?

The Guide to Trouble-Free Pool Maintenance

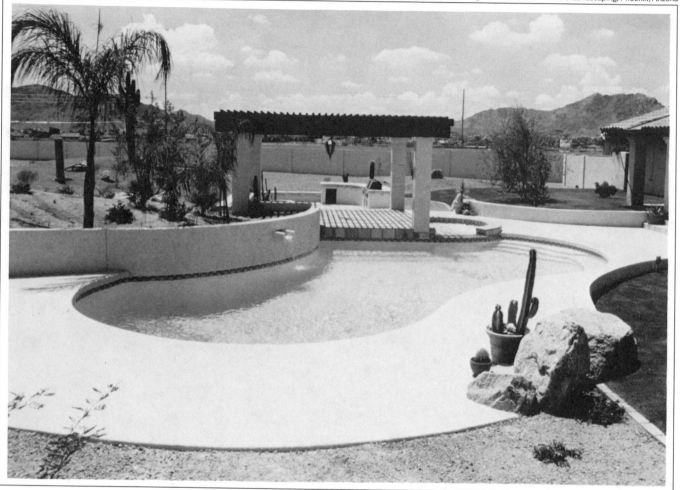

What Color Is Your
Swimming Pool?

The Guide to Trouble-Free Pool Maintenance

John M.O'Keefe

STOREY

STOREY COMMUNICATIONS, INC.
POWNAL, VERMONT

The mission of Storey Communications is to serve our customers by publishing practical information that encourages personal independence in harmony with the environment.

Design by Andrea Gray
Typesetting by Quad Left Graphics, Burlington, Vermont

Garden Way Publishing was founded in 1973 as part of the Garden Way Incorporated Group of Companies, dedicated to bringing gardening information and equipment to as many people as possible. Today the name "Garden Way Publishing" is licensed to Storey Communications, Inc., in Pownal, Vermont. For a complete list of Garden Way Publishing titles, call 1-800-827-8673. Garden Way Incorporated manufactures products in Troy, New York, under the Troy-Bilt® brand including garden tillers, chipper/shredders, mulching mowers, sicklebar mowers, and tractors. For information on any Garden Way Incorporated product, please call 1-800-345-4454.

Printed in the United States by Capital City Press
Seventeenth printing, August 1995

EDITOR'S NOTE

This book is intended to help, advise, guide, and introduce you to pool maintenance. It is **not** a repair manual, nor is it intended to be. If you find yourself in a position — even after following the information given herein — with water that is uncomfortable to swim in, or mechanical components that will not operate properly, it will probably be best for you and your pool system to call in the qualified services of a professional pool service company or repairman. The best advice we can give you is to establish a good and trustful relationship with a pool serviceman: one person who can be counselor, advisor, and repairman. You do the same thing for your pets and your car; take the time and make the effort to find a pool maintenance company or serviceman that you are comfortable with.

In order to do a good job of maintaining your pool system, you will need to be fairly vigilant about performing the tests and tasks outlined in the pages that follow. Pool maintenance is not without its drudgery, but if it provides you with a pool full of clean and sparkling water, then it will have been well worth the effort.

The information in this book is true and complete to the best of our knowledge. All recommendations are made without guarantee on the part of the author or Storey Communications, Inc. The author and publisher disclaim all liability incurred with the use of this information.

Contents

ACKNOWLEDGMENTS

I would like to thank and acknowledge the following individuals and organizations for their contributions to this book:

J. J. Tepas, a private pool product consultant, for his invaluable contribution to the section on water chemistry. For 30 years he was a consulting scientist with Olin Chemical, and has made major research and application contributions to the science of pool water chemistry, particularly in the area of pool water balancing.

Harry Clinton, of The Wet Institute for his invaluable contribution to the section on filters, pumps, and motors. The Wet Institute is an organization of professional pool builders specializing in educational pool dealer builder expansion programs.

And the National Spa & Pool Institute for their contributions of photographs and materials—particularly on pool safety and pool construction standards.

INTRODUCTION

Presumably you've got a swimming pool or intend to get one soon. Whether your pool has just been installed or you've had it for years, your enjoyment, pride of ownership, and even your investment depends on one basic factor — clean, healthful, sparkling water. That's the whole purpose of pumps, filters, cleaning systems, and pool chemicals. The point is this: How do you keep the pool and its water clean and healthy without spending a fortune on maintenance?

Perhaps your pool is not as clean as it should or could be? Is the water cloudy? Does algae sprout on the walls and bottom with annoying regularity? Are there streaks or stains marring the finish, odd smells, corroding plaster, skin and eye reactions, or rapid deterioration of pipes and equipment? These are hardly optimum conditions! They are evidence of inadequate, incorrect, or nonexistent water treatment or faulty mechanical systems. All of them, though, are easily corrected without major effort and expense if you take a little time to understand what a pool is, how it operates, and what you can reasonably do when things go wrong. That is the purpose of this book.

You can, of course, simply hand the whole job over to a pool service company, but presumably you're reading this book because you'd like to save some money by taking care of the pool yourself. Even if you prefer to let someone else do it, it's a smart idea to know something about the pool and its systems, so you can understand exactly why and for what a service company is billing you.

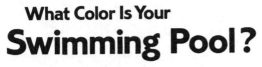

What Color Is Your
Swimming Pool?
The Guide to Trouble-Free Pool Maintenance

1 • Basic Pool Types and Construction

Continuing technological advances in pool construction materials and design have brought pool ownership within the reach of even the tightest family recreation budget. Today, you can get an above-ground pool kit for less than $500, but if you want it professionally installed, you can expect to pay more than twice as much. Prices for traditional in-ground pools range from $8,000 to $18,000 for a medium-size pool. The price you pay varies dramatically, depending on what type, size, shape, materials, and landscaping you want.

As with any investment, shopping around will get you the most value for your dollar. For those interested in buying a new pool, or replacing an existing older pool, I strongly suggest you contact the National Spa & Pool Institute, an industry organization for pool builders and suppliers with programs to help pool buyers avoid potential pitfalls and get the best value for their money. The NSPI has free brochures on pool planning, landscaping, energy saving, and pool buying. For a list of these and other available publications, write to NSPI, Publications Department, 2111 Eisenhower Avenue, Alexandria, Virginia 22314.

The purpose of this chapter is to explain briefly the various pool types on the market and their construction features. These differences do have some bearing on maintenance and cleaning procedures, which is the primary focus of this book.

In-Ground Pools

The most popular type of in-ground pool for reasons of economy and maintenance is the *vinyl-liner pool*. As with a concrete pool, a hole is dug and the rough plumbing is installed. A tough vinyl liner is then dropped into place, supported by a frame of aluminum, steel, plastic, masonry block, or wood. Tears in the liner can be repaired easily, often without draining the pool. Properly maintained, the liner can last up to 10 years before it needs replacing. Modern vinyl-liner pools are exceptionally durable and good-looking. Most come in a wide range of pre-formed sizes and shapes, but some manufacturers also offer custom pool shapes.

The most popular in-ground pool is the *Gunite* or Shotcrete pool. If you want an unusual pool shape, this is the one you need. A concrete mixture, called Gunite or Shotcrete,

POOL CONSTRUCTION METHODS

SPRAYED CONCRETE POOL

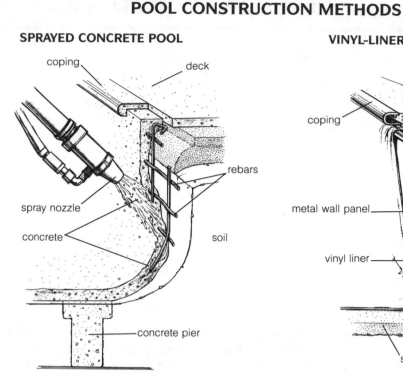

coping
deck
rebars
spray nozzle
concrete
soil
concrete pier

A wet or almost-dry concrete mixture is sprayed through a hose by intense air pressure onto a system of rebars (steel reinforcing rods) which form the pool site and shape.

VINYL-LINER POOL, METAL WALLS

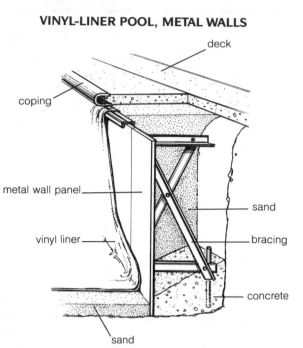

deck
coping
metal wall panel
sand
vinyl liner
bracing
concrete
sand

A durable vinyl liner is applied against a series of fitted metal wall panels that are supported with sand and bracing.

ONE-PIECE FIBERGLASS POOL

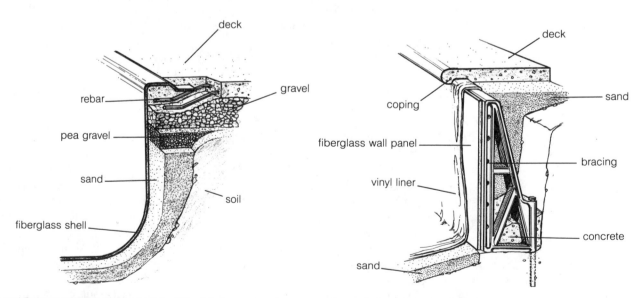

deck
rebar
gravel
pea gravel
sand
soil
fiberglass shell

A preformed fiberglass shell is lifted from a truck into the excavation site, and carefully backfilled with sand to assure that there are no gaps which could damage the shell when it is filled with water.

VINYL-LINER POOL, FIBERGLASS WALLS

deck
sand
coping
fiberglass wall panel
bracing
vinyl liner
concrete
sand

The structure and procedure is much the same as for vinyl-liner pools with metal walls, except that fiberglass panels have a greater resistance to deterioration from moisture and other elements.

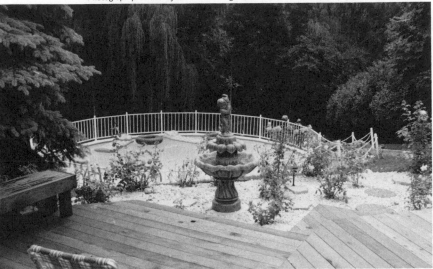

This vinyl-liner pool combines the best features of in-ground and above-ground construction.

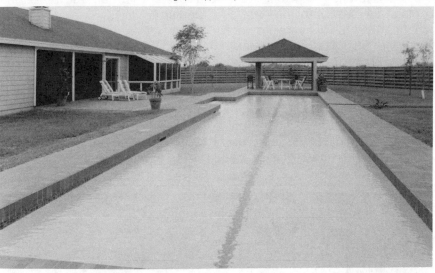

Lap pools have gained in popularity — due in part to the health revival and more attractive contemporary designs such as this Gunite pool.

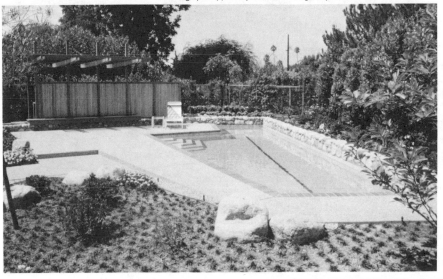

A Gunite pool, like the one here, gives you the design flexibility to suit a number of recreational needs.

is pneumatically applied to steel reinforcing rods and finished with a fine coat of plaster. The pool's thick concrete shell helps it to withstand frost pressures in cooler climates, and it rarely requires structural repairs. The primary advantage of a Gunite or Shotcrete pool is that it can be custom-designed in almost any shape you desire. Price can vary considerably depending on such factors as which part of the country you live in, soil and drainage problems, volume of pools built at that time, and difficulty with the weather.

A third option for an in-ground pool is fiberglass. You can buy these as a preformed shell in a variety of sizes and shapes, but you must have sufficient clearance room for a crane to place the shell into the excavation. Another type of fiberglass pool consists of fiberglass sidewalls and a concrete or vinyl bottom. These pools offer a greater variety of sizes and shapes than the one-piece, molded-fiberglass pools. The primary advantage of fiberglass is that it is easy to maintain, and the smooth surface makes algae re-

moval easy. Older pools can be resurfaced with fiberglass and various other coatings.

Above-Ground Pools

For those on a tight budget, an above-ground pool is the answer. Basically, it consists of a metal structural shell with a vinyl liner. These pools are generally restricted to round, oval, and rectangular shapes. The frame is usually aluminum or steel. If you haven't seen a well-designed above-ground pool, you might be in for a surprise. With landscaping around the pool, they can be equally as attractive and functional as their in-ground counterparts. They can also be set into sloping ground by excavating so that the water level almost reaches the ground level on the uphill side. Many models come in "kits" that can be assembled by two or three people over a weekend, using basic household tools. Adding a deck and other accessories can make an above-ground pool an attractive addition to the home.

If you haven't seen a well-designed above-ground pool, you might be in for a surprise.

Photograph is supplied by the NSPI. Design: Les Embellissements Paysager Laval; Chomeday, Quebec

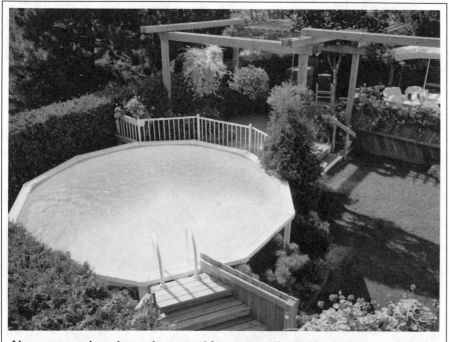

Above-ground pools can be every bit as appealing as in-ground pools when attention is given to the complete pool landscaping area.

Although this is a pool maintenance and not a construction book, all prospective pool builders should become educated in the terminology and specificities of the industry.

In particular:

- Your local town or city hall will tell you what the setback, fencing, and insurance requirements will be. While you're there, ask how long it will take to get a building permit.
- Get the names of reputable pool installation companies from friends, neighbors, and acquaintances. Get at least three estimates, and determine exactly what the work on the estimate represents. Have these companies supply you with a list of clients who live nearby. Hopefully you can either speak to these customers or inspect the work of the company yourself.
- Do not sign any contract until every clause has been made clear to you.
- Write to the NSPI for their publications on pool planning, building, and a list of pool installation companies which are accepted members of the NSPI. NSPI membership is generally an indication of a pool company's success and integrity.

2 • Water

Water is the most common substance on earth. Without it, there would be no life. In fact, two-thirds of the human body consists of water. Water has also been called the universal solvent, and for good reason. It is the master sculptor of the earth: rain washes soil into rivers, oceans carve away cliffs and build shorelines, and rivers cut through rock, carving out valleys and gorges. However, water in its natural state is seldom free of minerals, bacteria, or unpleasant tastes and odors. Even treated water from the tap in your home, if not treated, becomes an excellent breeding ground for bacteria and algae. Water has one other quality that is important as it relates to pool maintenance: it has the ability to corrode, dissolve, and calcify a wide range of substances. In as little as 5 years, ordinary drinking water can corrode large concrete storage tanks to such a point that they become virtually useless. This is why certain chemicals are added to pool water to prevent corrosion of pool walls and equipment, and to avoid cloudiness, scaling, and calcification. This process is know as *balancing the water*.

An Introduction to Water Chemistry

Basically, a molecule of water consists of one atom of oxygen and two atoms of hydrogen, bound together by shared electrons (the negative and positive electrical charges that bind atoms together). When atoms become negatively or positively charged through combination and a subsequent exchange of electrons, they are thereafter referred to as *ions*.

In nature only about two molecules of water per billion undergo a change: one hydrogen atom breaks away from the rest of the molecule forming a positively-charged *hydrogen ion* and a negatively-charged *hydroxide ion*. In a given volume of water, although most of the water exists as water molecules, some hydrogen ions and some hydroxide ions are also present. It is the proportion of these hydrogen and hydroxide ions to the rest of the water molecules that determines whether water is *acidic* or *alkaline*. And this can be easily measured. Although testing pool water to determine

It is the proportion of these hydrogen and hydroxide ions to the rest of the water molecules that determines whether water is *acidic* or *alkaline*.

6

whether it is acidic or alkaline is the single most important step for satisfactory water treatment, a number of other tests are also necessary. These will be described on the pages that follow.

The pH Scale

The system devised by chemists for indicating the acidity or alkalinity of water involves a scale of numbers, called the *pH scale* (pH stands for potential hydrogen). The scale runs from 1 to 14, with 7 representing water which is neutral—neither acidic nor alkaline. Numbers below 7 indicate a greater concentration of hydrogen ions, or an acidic condition; numbers above 7 indicate an alkaline condition. The human body, for instance, has a pH factor of 7.3 to 7.5—slightly alkaline.

The cause of most swimming pool water problems is incorrect pH levels. If you swim in water with a pH of below 7.0, you may experience eye and skin irritation. When pH is too low, the water can eat away plaster, tile grout and cement, metal pipes and equipment, and cause swimming discomfort. When pH is too high, the water can deposit chemicals such as calcium carbonate that produces scale on pool walls and inside pipes, pumps, filters, and other equipment, causing numerous problems such as restricted water flow and poor filtration. Swimming pool water is best for its users and the pool system at a pH between 7.2 and 7.6. The aim of balancing pool water is to main-

tain the water so that neither of these conditions occur. How to go about doing that is the subject of the next chapter.

The Need for Sterilizers

In addition to controlling the chemical balance of pool water, sterilization is also required. Warm swimming pool water is a natural breeding ground for bacteria, algae, and other organic contaminants. Swimmers introduce bacteria, dirt, germs, skin particles, body oils, urine, and other body excretions into the water. This pollution will reduce the clarity of the water, change its color, and give it an unpleasant taste and odor. Such water is also a distinct hazard to health, unless it is correctly sanitized.

Sterilizing chemicals such as chlorine or bromine are added to pool water to kill bacteria, algae, and germs. Adequate dosages of pool-sterilizing chemicals (chlorine sanitizers, for instance) also oxidize the dead organic matter. That is, they chemically "burn" it up so you're not left with a pool full of dead organic matter.

The main point to remember is that correctly balancing the pool water will not only protect the pool and equipment and make swimming more pleasant, but will also enhance and extend the killing effect of pool-sterlizing chemicals. It is a waste of time and money to sanitize and disinfect a pool full of unbalanced water—to avoid this situation, read ahead.

> Numbers below 7 indicate a greater concentration of hydrogen ions, or an acidic condition; numbers above 7 indicate an alkaline condition.

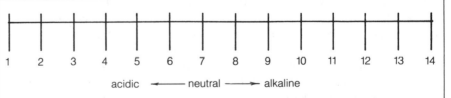

acidic ◄——— neutral ———► alkaline

The pH scale was devised to calculate water's acidity or alkalinity. Seven represents water that has a neutral chemical composition; numbers below 7 indicates acidic water; numbers above 7 indicate alkaline water.

3 • Water Treatment

Incorrect or inadequate water treatment can create serious problems and needless expense. I wish I could tell you there is a simple technique that takes only a few minutes of your time each week, but there isn't. Proper treatment requires that you invest a little time to gain an understanding of what's involved. You can then expect to spend some time each week (possibly up to 3 hours) during the swimming season on water treatment and routine maintenance chores, such as vacuuming the pool and cleaning out leaves and other debris that gather in the pump-strainer and skimmer baskets. Screened or otherwise enclosed pools considerably reduce the need for such maintenance. If this kind of maintenance is neither possible nor acceptable, you can expect to pay a pool service company to do it for you. In order to adequately evaluate your own capabilities or those of a pool service company, it will help to know the basics of water treatment. One way or another, it will prove valuable to understand the process by which pool water is made swimmable.

The work involved in doing your own water treatment is not back-breaking by any means and can actually be gratifying and quite enjoyable. Among the rewards are the satisfaction and peace of mind that come with knowing your pool and equipment are functioning as they should, and that unseen problems are not setting you up for expensive repair bills.

What is the goal of water treatment? Sparkling clean, hazard-free water that is not so acidic as to irritate your skin and eyes and corrode expensive pool equipment, nor so alkaline that it is uncomfortable to swim in and forms destructive scale on pool surfaces and equipment. Despite what you may have been told or read in advertisements, there is no standard water treatment procedure for all pools. Although there are broad parameters that may be followed, water treatment can be different for every pool. There are wide regional differences in water characteristics: acidity, hardness or softness, concentration of dissolved minerals, and the amount of bacteria and algae present in the water are all factors to consider in its treatment. Atmospheric and wind-borne pollutants also affect the water, as does the amount of use the pool gets, the personal hygiene of those swimming in it, sunlight, air and water temperature, the type of chemicals you employ, and the efficiency and length of time the filter system is in operation. If you understand the basic principles discussed here, you should be able to tailor your water treatment program to suit your particular situation and any water peculiarities.

HOW MUCH WATER IN YOUR POOL?

Before tackling any water treatment, you have to know how much water your pool contains so that you can correctly calculate the amount of treatment chemicals you will need. Below are equations to help you calculate the approximate gallonage for pools of various shapes. Chemical containers list how many ounces or pounds to use per thousand gallons of water.

Circular pools. For pools with straight sides, multiply the pool diameter by itself (square the diameter), then multiply that amount by its average depth in feet. Multiply the result by 5.9.

Oval pools. For pools with straight sides, multiply full width by full length, by average depth in feet. Then multiply by 5.9.

Rectangular pools. Multiply the length by the width by the average depth in feet. Then multiply by 7.5.

Irregular pools. Figuring these are a bit more difficult. If you cannot get the gallonage from your pool contractor, you can get an approximate figure by dividing the overall shape into smaller geometric forms—squares, rectangles, circles, or ovals—and figuring the gallonage in each. Then add them together.

Illustration by Wanda Harper

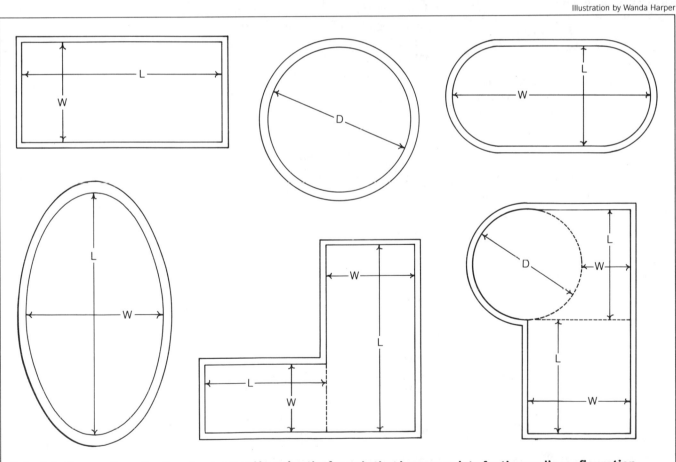

Calculate the number of gallons in your pool by using the formula that is appropriate for the pool's configuration.

DISINFECTANTS

In order to assure cleanliness and freedom from germs and algae, the proper addition of disinfectants to the pool water is crucial. These materials influence pH and other indicators, yet their effectiveness can be hampered if water is not properly balanced. This section will discuss your chemical options and the procedures that will clean and sanitize your pool water: iodine, bromine, chlorine, and superchlorination.

Iodine. Iodine is an effective germicide, but it has not gained widespread acceptance, mainly because it needs careful regulation, and too much can discolor the water. It is not recommended for use by the occasional or casual maintenance person or pool owner.

Bromine. Bromine in stick and powder form is making some inroads as a pool sanitizer. It chemically reacts with water to form hypobromous acid and hypobromide ions. Hypobromous acid is the more effective sanitizer. As the water pH reaches higher levels, the active hypobromous acid decreases, which reduces its sanitizing effectiveness, but the reduction is not as severe as it is with chlorine. Perhaps the main advantage of bromine is that it doesn't cause eye irritation or odor problems. The disadvantages of bromine include higher cost, the need for a higher free bromine residual in the water than with chlorine, and the fact that bromine is not stabilized to sunlight, which increases the loss of bromine in the water.

Chlorine. This is by far the most popular and widely used pool disinfectant, as well as being the standard disinfecting agent recommended by health experts and pool specialists. Available in gas, liquid, powder, and tablet form, chlorine can quickly reduce organic matter and disease-causing organisms.

The use of chlorine gas is restricted to professional application. It is dangerous to handle and requires trained supervision and expensive equipment to dispense it safely into water. For this reason, all future mention of "chlorination" refers to the use of dry or liquid chlorine sanitizers.

Liquid chlorine (sodium hypochlorite) is an inexpensive and popular form of chlorine. It disperses quickly in water and leaves no residue. It does, however, raise the pH and alkalinity of the water and requires careful handling to avoid skin injury or damage to clothes. Also, it can deteriorate if stored too long. The concentration of liquid chlorine varies regionally, but it is usually sold at a concentration of between 10 to 15 percent. Household bleach contains only about 5 percent chlorine.

Chlorine can also be purchased in dry form as *calcium hypochlorite, lithium hypochlorite,* and as *chlorinated isocyanurics.* Calcium hypochorite granules, sticks, and tablets contain about 65 percent pure chlorine. It resists deterioration and is

Illustrations by Chrysalis Design Group

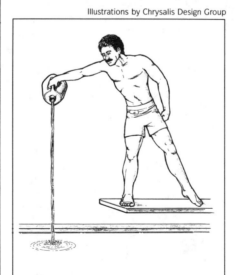

Pour liquid chlorine into the pool so that it will disperse quickly in the water; the easiest way to do this is to pour the chlorine as far away from the edges as possible. Be careful not to let the chlorine splash onto your skin or clothing.

In order to assure cleanliness and freedom from germs and algae, the proper addition of disinfectants to the pool water is crucial.

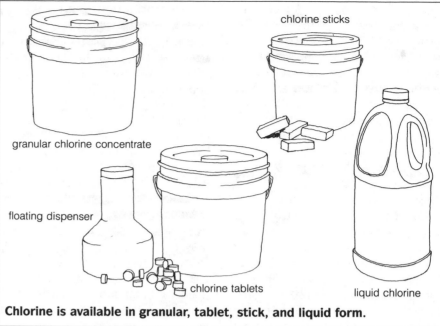

granular chlorine concentrate

chlorine sticks

floating dispenser

chlorine tablets

liquid chlorine

Chlorine is available in granular, tablet, stick, and liquid form.

When dispensing dry chlorine *always* add it to the water, and not vice versa. Use a nonmetal container for mixing.

easy to handle and store. You can avoid most of the cloudiness sometimes obtained with granular calcium hypochlorite by mixing 8 ounces with 10 quarts of water in a nonmetallic container (always follow product instructions first). Lithium hypochlorite comes in granular form, and because it is less alkaline than calcium hypochlorite, there is not as much pH adjustment necessary. Chlorinated isocyanurics dissolve easily, have slightly greater resistance to dissipation by sunlight, do not increase calcium hardness, and do not substantially affect the pH level. But they should be used only according to the directions provided because they can give off dangerous fumes.

When dispensing dry chlorine *always* add it to the water, and not vice versa. Use a nonmetal container for mixing, unless specified otherwise in the chlorine instructions. Stir for about 30 seconds, then set aside out of the sun for 30 minutes to allow the solids to settle. Then pour the clear liquid into the pool and discard the sediment. Sticks and tablets are applied through dispensers plumbed into the water-inlet lines of the pool. The chlorine is released gradually as the flow of water dissolves the tablets. There are also floating dispensers that achieve the same result.

No matter what form of chlorine is used, when it is added to water hypochlorite ions and hypochlorous acid are formed. Hypochlorous acid is the active sanitizing agent that kills bacteria and algae, removes odors, and destroys organic contaminants. The amount of desirable hypochlorous acid produced from a certain dosage of chlorine sanitizer is determined by the pH of the water. For this reason, it is usually wiser to test and adjust the pH *before* adding chlorine to the water.

When chlorine is added to pool water, a certain portion is consumed in the process of destroying bacteria, algae, and other organic contaminants. The amount of chlorine consumed in this initial reaction is known as the *chlorine demand* of the pool. The amount of active sanitizer remaining after this demand has been satisfied is known as the *chlorine residual*. A certain chlorine residual must be maintained in order to destroy bacteria, algae, or viruses introduced into the water by swimmers or through the air by dust, rain, and other sources. You can use an inexpensive, basic test kit to determine the chlorine residual in the pool. The chlorine residual in a pool should be maintained between 1.0 and 1.5 parts per million (or ppm). In this range, chlorine controls organisms injurious to health and provides a safety margin against incoming contamination.

It is a common misunderstanding that if the water has a strong chlorine odor, too much chlorine has been added. On the contrary, this is an indicator of *too little* free residual chlorine in the water. Pool water contains ammonia which it gets from fertilizers blown or washed in from lawns and gardens, urine, and natural body oils and perspiration. Ammonia reacts with chlorine to form *chloramine* (combined chlorine), which is the major cause of burning eyes, skin irritation, and the unpleasant chlorine odor. The odor is particularly pungent if pH is low. Chlorine in an uncombined or free state is practically odorless. So, when people start complaining of burning eyes and that "chlorine smell," realize it is because there is *too little free residual chlorine* in the water, not too much.

Sunlight dissipates chlorine. If you are going to use a chlorine sanitizer that is not stabilized to reduce the effects of sunlight, you may need to add a stabilizer that will lessen the effect of sunlight on chlorine dissipation. Ask your pool supply dealer at the beginning of the season what kind of stabilizer you will need for the chlorine you use, and how much stabilizer to add.

In most outdoor pools with stabilized water, the use of chlorine three or four times a week during the swimming season should keep the residual at a safe level. But the water should always be tested for residual chlorine before adding chlorine to the water so you know how much to add. Therefore, test and adjust the pH to correct levels before adding the chlorine.

Superchlorination. Superchlorination is simply an extra dose of chlorine—a kind of shock treatment—to burn out bacteria, algae, nitrogen compounds, and especially ammonia, all or some of which have not been eliminated by routine chlorination. Three to five times the normal dose of chlorine is added to the pool as directed on the product instructions, or as recommended by a pool service professional. Increased bathing loads and increased algae growth during summer months, when unheated water may reach a temperature of 85°F (30°C) or more, may make superchlorination necessary. You may need to superchlorinate when bad odors or algae (green or colored water) are visible, when bathers complain of eye irritation, or after the pool has had a period of heavy use.

The best time to superchlorinate is after sundown, to avoid chlorine waste through dissipation by the sun's ultraviolet rays. You can do it at other times, but do not allow anyone to use the pool until the residual chlorine level drops back to normal (which, in most pools, is below 3.0 ppm). The product directions should give you the amount of time needed before you can safely use the pool again. If this information is not provided, ask a pool service company how long you have to wait before swimming can be allowed. If at any time between scheduled superchlorination treatments, the chlorine residual drops to 0, the water should be superchlorinated promptly. A reading of 0 is often, in fact, below 0, which means that some chlorine demand has accumulated in the water, and bacteria and algae growth will develop rapidly. In hot weather, a residual reading of 0 can turn the pool water cloudy and green within a day or two.

One word of caution: don't superchlorinate when the pH level is low (overacid). If you do, any copper dissolved from the pool equipment or

When people start complaining of burning eyes and that "chlorine smell," realize it is because there is *too little free residual chlorine* in the water, not too much.

The best time to superchlorinate is after sundown, to avoid chlorine waste through dissipation by the sun's ultraviolet rays.

plumbing by the acidic water may be oxidized by the large dose of chlorine and cause black stains on the pool finish.

POOL WATER TEST KITS

Before going any further, a word about water test kits is in order. You can buy simple, inexpensive test kits from pool supply stores or pool builders and dealers. My advice is to buy a kit that measures not only chlorine residual and pH, but also the amount of total alkalinity and calcium hardness of the pool water. Such measurements are vital to attain correctly balanced water. If you have difficulty finding a kit that measures calcium hardness, most pool supply stores will measure the calcium hardness for you if you bring a quart sample of pool water. Be sure to use a completely clean container for any sample of water.

The tests for chlorine residual and pH consist of filling a small tube to the indicated level with pool water and adding measured drops of chemical reagents. These reagents react with chemicals in the water that will color it. The treated water is then compared to a standard color chart to determine chlorine and pH levels. Always take the water sample from at least 12 inches below the water level. Many substances tend to float in the top layer of water and these can give false readings. When you shake or invert the test kit don't put your finger over the top of the tube because body acid can also affect the reading. Judge the color of the sample against a light background (preferably white) and try to use the same background each time, to avoid variances in readings on bright or cloudy days. Always rinse the sample tube after use and never use it for any other type of solution. For best results, replace the chemicals in the test kit once a year.

With a new pool, you should test for chlorine daily during the first

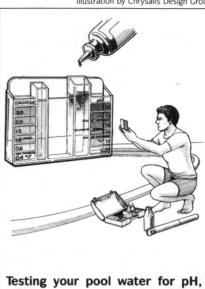

Testing your pool water for pH, chlorine residual, total alkalinity, and calcium hardness is an important part of pool maintenance. Chemical reagents are added to a water sample that will give you an indication of the water's condition and what course of treatment will then be necessary.

month, then two or three times weekly. Frequent testing and pH adjustments for a new pool, particularly a plaster pool, is very important. Fresh plaster needs time to harden. You need to keep the pH around 7.4 to 7.6 during this time. If the pH drops too low (becomes too acidic) the water will get the calcium it requires from the new plaster. The pH should be tested once or even twice a day in a new pool, and adjusted to the 7.4 to 7.6 range.

Another option is to bring a sample of your pool water to a pool supply dealer once or twice a year to obtain a computerized printout with the chemical composition (pH, chlorine residual, calcium hardness, total alkalinity) of your water. From this reading, you will have a fairly accurate analysis of what will be needed to bring your water into balance. If you live in an area with a limited swimming season, take in a water sample about a week or ten days after you have opened up the pool.

Always take the water sample from at least 12 inches below the water level. Many substances tend to float in the top layer of water and these can give false readings.

THE IMPORTANCE OF pH

Earlier, it was recommended that you not add chlorine to the pool until you've checked and adjusted the pH level. The reason for this lies in the chemistry of water and what happens to chemicals in pool water. Chlorine, as stated earlier, forms hypochlorite ions and hypochlorous acid when added to water. It is the hypochlorous acid (also known as free chlorine) that does most of the disinfecting work. The proportion of useful hypochlorous acid and the not-so-useful hypochlorite ions is determined by pH. For instance, at a pH of 7.0, the presence of hypochlorous acid in the water can be as high as 80 percent, with only 20 percent present as ineffective hypochlorite ions. When pH is allowed to drop to 7.0 the water will be too acidic for comfortable swimming, and at this level, it will attack pool surfaces and equipment. The recommended pH range for pool water lies between 7.2 and 7.6; this allows the most economical use of chlorine without putting the water out of balance. If the water is allowed to reach a pH of 8.0 or higher (and it is not unusual to find this in private pools) you will have to maintain two to three times the chlorine residual to produce the same amount of sanitizing hypochlorous acid ions.

The pH is controlled by adding either acid or alkali products. Acid is used to lower the pH, alkali to increase it. You can use liquid *muriatic acid* or dry *sodiuim bisulphate* to lower pH, both of which are available at pool supply stores. Make sure the acid mixes well with the water by dispensing it around the pool. The filter pump should be turned on to circulate the acid more thoroughly throughout the pool. Don't add acid through the skimmer—it can damage pipes, fittings, and equipment. Handle acid very carefully so that it doesn't burn you or damage anything. It is advisable to wear goggles and gloves when dispensing acid, and wash any spills off clothing or decking immediately. Sodium bisulphate is a dry acid which is also used to lower pH. Follow the instructions on the label exactly to ensure that the proper amount is administered to disinfect and maintain water balance. And remember that the amounts of acid given on the product label to lower the pH are only approximate. Experiment with various dosages to achieve the results that are best for your pool.

If the pH reading is too low (below 7.2), it can be raised by adding soda ash (sodium carbonate) to the water. Soda ash can be purchased at pool supply stores. You can also use plain household baking soda (sodium bicarbonate) to raise pH, but you may need to add quite a bit and it will increase the alkalinity level as well. This, of course, can be a good thing if the alkalinity is too low, but not otherwise. Alkaline compounds used to raise pH levels usually contain a printed chart on the package that lists the approximate dosages needed to raise the pH by a specified amount. It should be

Illustration by Chrysalis Design Group

Liquid and dry acid is very toxic — handle it carefully. Pour it close to the water to prevent splashing and away from the pool's edges to allow maximum dispersion.

The recommended pH range for pool water lies between 7.2 and 7.6; this allows the most economical use of chlorine without putting the water out of balance.

Don't add acid through the skimmer — it can damage pipes, fittings, and equipment.

The amount of calcium in the water determines whether it is hard or soft. With too little calcium, the water becomes soft — corrosive to plaster and equipment. The presence of too much calcium can lead to the formation of scale on pool surfaces and inside pipes, heater coils, and filters.

Cyanuric Acid 50 ideal

Over 40 takes pts away from alkal.

clear by this point that pH and total alkalinity are closely related, so total alkalinity is the next subject for discussion.

Total Alkalinity *weekly*

Total alkalinity (or TA) refers to the total amount of all alkali compounds (soluble salts) in the water. These include bicarbonates, carbonates, hydroxides, and other alkali compounds. The water's total alkalinity determines its resistance to large fluctuations in pH levels. Total alkalinity of water supplies vary considerably in different areas of the country, and even between adjacent communities. Like other water tests, testing for total alkalinity consists of a simple color test, using reagents and a sample of pool water.

When the total alkalinity is high, the pH tends to remain high also. The acid used to lower pH will also lower the total alkalinity for a short time, but because of the high total alkalinity present, the pH will generally bounce back up again. The range of desirable total alkalinity for pool water varies between *80* to *130* ppm, depending on the particular conditions existing in your pool, and to some extent, on the type of sanitizer used. The way to get it right for your pool is to watch the pH level. If the pH tends to go up after adding acid to lower it, the total alkalinity is too high. If the pH tends to drop below the desirable range, the alkalinity is too low. When the alkalinity is just right for your pool conditions, the pH level will practically stabilize; that is, it will rise or fall at a much slower rate. As a rule of thumb, if the pH in your pool tends to rise, aim for a total alkalinity of 50 to 80 ppm. If the pH tends to drop, aim for a total alkalinity of 80 to 125 ppm.

In general terms, if the total alkalinity reading is too high, add the specified amount of muriatic acid for your size pool to bring it within the accepted range. You may have to repeat muriatic acid dosages several times before the TA comes into an acceptable range. Remember that the acid will also lower the pH, so if it dips below the 7.2 level, add soda ash to bring the pH back up.

If the total alkalinity reading is too low, use sodium bicarbonate to raise it. Don't use soda ash to raise alkalinity because it will send the pH skyrocketing. One of the nice things about sodium bicarbonate is that it can only raise the pH of the pool to its own maximum pH level (8.3) no matter how much you put in. If both the pH and total alkalinity are too low, first increase the total alkalinity to the correct range. Often, this will also bring the pH up to an acceptable level without further treatment.

Calcium Hardness *monthly*

Another factor to consider in water treatment is calcium hardness, which is a measure of the amount of dissolved calcium compounds in the water. The amount of calcium in the water determines whether it is hard or soft. With too little calcium, the water becomes soft — corrosive to plaster and equipment. The presence of too much calcium can lead to the formation of scale on pool surfaces and inside pipes, heater coils, and filters. The reason for this is that water of a given temperature and pH can only hold a certain concentration of calcium carbonates in solution.

There is no definitive calcium hardness level. Most pool experts recommend a calcium hardness of at least 200 ppm, but no higher than 500 ppm. The calcium hardness level can be raised by adding calcium chloride, but before you try to adjust the calcium hardness get the advice and recommendation of a pool service professional. Calcium hardness tends not to be a priority in water treatment, even among many pool service companies. However, when it comes to balancing the water — which is strongly recommended — calcium hardness is an important factor.

Cynauric Aeg

5/8 210 T

80 Al

WATER BALANCING

This section brings all the factors previously discussed together: chlorination, pH, total alkalinity, and calcium hardness.

Just as water always tries to balance its level physically, it also tries to balance itself chemically. Chemical balance means maintaining the essential ingredient of calcium carbonate at or above the demand of the water for this ingredient, so that the water has no desire to get this or other chemical compounds from the pool cement, plaster, tile grout, or from the equipment. Water's "hunger" for calcium carbonate can damage or impede the operation of the pool system, but this situation can be avoided by proper water balancing. To successfully balance your pool water, you will need to bring the pH, TA, and calcium hardness into alignment.

What must be clearly understood is that the amount of calcium the water needs or demands, *depends* on the water's pH and total alkalinity levels. A typical water balancing scale based on the Langelier Index (Figure 3.1) is shown on page 17. As you can see from this simplified scale, there is not one set of figures for theoretically balanced water, but hundreds or even thousands. For instance, if the water is at a pH of 7.4, position a ruler or straightedge to intersect the center column where 7.4 is marked, By moving the ruler up or down, you can get any number of combinations of total alkalinity and calcium hardness that will indicate balanced water. But note that if the pH is 7.6 and total alkalinity is 100, you must either raise or lower the calcium hardness to 200 to get balanced water. Similarly, if the calcium hardness is 400 and pH is 7.6, then the total alkalinity must be adjusted to about 50 ppm.

From this scale, you can see why knowing and adjusting only the pH level and the total alkalinity may not give you balanced water. At a pH of 7.4 and a total alkalinity of 100 ppm, the calcium hardness must be adjusted to 300 ppm or the water will be out of balance. If, in this case, the calcium hardness were 200 ppm (pH and TA being the same), guess where the water will get the other 100 ppm of calcium carbonate? The surfaces of a plaster pool would be its preferred source. If denied this, the water will do its best to digest any other materials with which it has contact.

The most constant factor in all this is the pH range you want to work with. The recommended range lies between 7.2 and 7.6. To balance the water in your pool, test the pH, total alkalinity, and calcium hardness. The most difficult level to reduce is calcium hardness. For this reason, it is simpler to take the calcium hardness reading (if in the recommended range) as a stable point and adjust the pH and total alkalinity to suit the calcium hardness level. But this is not a fixed rule by any means. Neither is the formula outlined above precise or foolproof. It you have trouble reaching a reasonable balance, get the counsel of a pool service person who may be aware of peculiarities or methods to assist you.

Once the water in your pool is balanced, it is much easier to maintain it that way than if the water is unbalanced, since you are giving the water what it wants naturally. But note that the balance can be upset by rain (changing the pH level), or the need for greater amounts of chlorine due to heavy pool activity. That is why pool water treatment should be part of a regular maintenance schedule. Regular water testing for free chlorine level, pH, and total alkalinity should be done twice a week during the summer months. Calcium hardness is relatively stable, but it should be checked at least monthly.

For those interested in a more detailed review of water balancing, I recommend the *HTH Water Book for*

Once the water in your pool is balanced, it is much easier to maintain it that way than if the water is unbalanced, since you are giving the water what it wants naturally. The balance can be upset by rain (changing the pH level), or the need for heavier amounts of chlorine due to heavy pool activity.

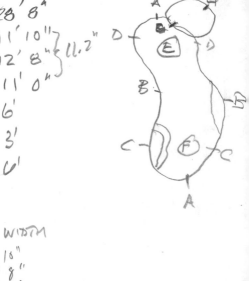

WHAT COLOR IS YOUR SWIMMING POOL?

A WATER BALANCING EXPERIMENT

Suppose you perform various tests on the chemical composition of your pool water and get the following readings: pH 7.6, total alkalinity 40, calcium hardness 220. Using Figure 3.1 draw a straight line between the total alkalinity and calcium hardness readings to show that for the water to be balanced, the pH must be raised to almost 8.0. A pH of 8.0 is far too high for swimming comfort and will increase the use of chlorine considerably. Keeping one end of the line on a calcium hardness factor of 225 ppm, bring the other end down to intersect at a more suitable pH level, such as 7.4. This shows that the total alkalinity should be brought up to around 130 ppm.

Take a moment to sit down and work this out on paper. From the charts supplied with the chemicals, you can find out how many pounds of sodium bicarbonate are needed to raise the alkalinity to the desired level. But remember, sodium bicarbonate will also increase the pH. Figure out how much acid is needed to bring the pH down to the desired 7.4 level. Write that down also. As stated earlier, acid will also lower the total alkalinity, which you do not want. To compensate for the acid, increase the amount of bicarbonate. These calculations are simple to do if you use the charts supplied with these chemicals.

Which chemical goes in first? Well, the pH is high, so add the acid first. Thoroughly mix it in a plastic bucket of water and either pour it around the perimeter of the pool or near an inlet where the filtered water returns into the pool, to ensure good mixing. Make sure the filter pump is running. On the other hand, if the pH is too low and has to be raised, you add the bicarbonate first, then the acid, because the water is already too acidic. The bicarbonate should be evenly distributed across the surface of the pool. Wait at least an hour before adding the acid. You can test pH again before adding the acid to check your calculations.

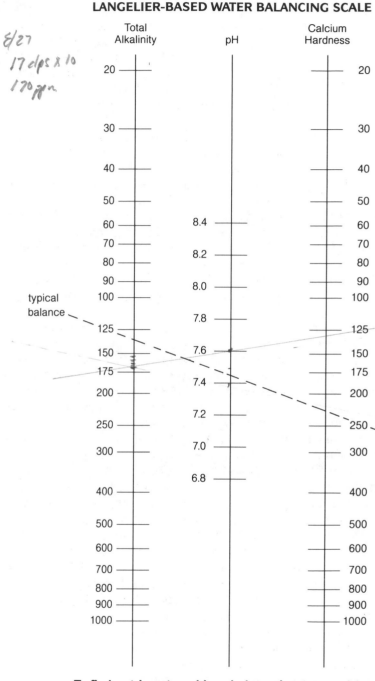

FIGURE 3.1:
LANGELIER-BASED WATER BALANCING SCALE

To find out how to achieve balanced water, position a ruler or straight edge to intersect at the approximate pH and calcium hardness readings of your pool water. This will give you the total alkalinity required to balance the water. The typical balance in the chart shows that with a pH of 7.4 and a calcium hardness of 225, total alkalinity should be 130 ppm.

Pool Professionals, written by J. J. Tepas, J. P. Fause, and R. L. Waldvogel, consulting scientists at Olin Corporation. To get a copy, write Olin Corporation, Consumer Products Department, 120 Long Ridge Road, Stamford, Connecticut 06904.

New Pools

Although reputable pool builders will fill new pools and supervise their initial treatment, it is advisable for the pool owner to understand why particular care is needed at this time, particularly if the pool is concrete surfaced with plaster or tile.

Iron, manganese, and/or metallic salts are present in the water in many localities. Even though the water is drinkable, these minerals can give it an unattractive color and stain pool surfaces. You would be well advised to have a sample of the water in your new pool tested for mineral content at a pool service center. Excessive amounts of these minerals in your water supply (above 0.2 ppm) may persuade you to take special precautions to prevent staining. If the iron level is 0.2 ppm or below, you can use one of a number of antistaining compounds available at a pool supply store. Follow the directions carefully.

If the iron level is 0.2 or above, and you don't have a diatomaceous earth (DE) filter, buy enough alum or other flocculent from your pool supply dealer to treat the amount of water in your pool. This normally works out to be about one pound of alum for each 5,000 gallons of water. *Flocculents* attract iron and other contaminants such as dirt into larger masses which then come out of suspension in the water and sink to the pool floor where they can be vacuumed or removed by the filter.

In a new pool, the pH must not be too low or too high. There is some disagreement among experts as to whether the pH should be adjusted before or after using alum. The consensus is to adjust the pH to about 7.6, then add the alum according to package directions. One effective way is to fill a burlap bag with the recommended amount of alum and tie it to a stick or pole; vigorously dunk the bag in the pool until most of the alum has been dissolved. The next step is to superchlorinate the pool. Superchlorination precipitates iron and other metal salts in the water, causing them to fall to the floor of the pool, so a flocculent may not be needed after all. Experiment: you'll know after performing this procedure once or twice whether a flocculent will be necessary or not. And ask several local pool installers what they recommend, based on their experience with the pools in your neighborhood.

After "floccing" or superchlorinating the pool, vacuum the pool walls and floor to remove precipitated iron. Set the vacuum control to route water directly to waste, so there is no risk that iron will be recirculated through the filter and back into the pool. The water should be clearing up nicely by now. If not, you will have to add more alum until a sparkling blue color is obtained. Regardless of whether you shut down the filter system while adding chlorine, or keep the filter running throughout, you should keep an eye on the filter gauge. Alum can quickly block a DE or cartridge filter so backwash the filter each time the gauge shows a differential of 5 to 7 pounds per square inch (or psi). Such a differential will probably occur every 2 hours during this process.

Test the pH often and don't let it fall below 7.2. When the iron salts have been precipitated and vacuumed to waste, and the water is clear, you can use a commercial stain inhibitor to handle iron present in the makeup or refill water.

For new pools in which iron in the water is not a problem, don't begin chlorination until the water has

Flocculents attract iron and other contaminants such as dirt into larger masses which then come out of suspension in the water and sink to the pool floor where they can be vacuumed, or removed by the filter.

> Keeping pH at acceptable levels and maintaining the recommended level of free chlorine will minimize the chances of algae growth.

reached the level of the pool's water-line tile. Adjust the water to the desired total alkalinity and calcium hardness levels before adding chlorine. New plastered concrete pools are filled as soon as the plaster "sets" because it must harden (cure) under water. Acid should be added to the water sparingly for the first 2 weeks; use the recommended dilution and distribute evenly, with the pool filter running. Most pool builders recommend the pH level for new plastered concrete pools be kept in the 7.6 to 7.8 range. Your builder should advise you on this because if you do not follow given specifications you may void any guarantee or the builder's liability for damage to the pool. Statements to this effect are usually written into standard pool contracts.

Daily brushing with a wall brush is recommended to remove the fine, cloudy sediment that builds up on the walls and floor of a new plastered concrete pool. This sediment is normal and will disappear in a few weeks as the surface hardens. Keep the filter system in operation during and after brushing. *Do not* use a vacuum or automatic pool cleaner at this time. The wheels can compress surface sediment into the pores of the walls and floor, which can form stain areas.

COMMON WATER PROBLEMS

This is the final section on water treatment: typical water problems and how to correct them. If you properly maintain the water, many of these problems may never arise because most of them are either caused by, or due in part to, unbalanced water. But stains, algae infestations, and other problems can occur despite your best efforts, so it is best to know how to cope with them.

> Once established, algae fosters the growth of bacteria.

Algae

Algae is one of the most resourceful and persistent forms of plant life. It can be free-floating in the water, or it can cling to walls, floor, and equipment. Nourished by sunlight and heat, algae thrives in water with a high pH level. If you see it in your pool, you had better take steps to eradicate it immediately, because it can cover the entire surface of your pool in a matter of hours. And, once established, algae fosters the growth of bacteria. If you ignore the warning signs and let algae get completely out of hand, chances are the pool will have to be drained, and the walls and floors scrubbed with full-strength chlorine. Algae can turn the pool water green, cloudy, and/or cause spots to form on the walls. One of the most frequent signs of algae growth is a sudden slipperiness on pool surfaces, particularly steps in the shallow end.

Keeping pH at acceptable levels and maintaining the recommended level of free chlorine will minimize the chances of algae growth. But if you skip a day or two of chlorination or don't compensate for a heavy weekend bathing load or extremely hot weather, algae may appear. Superchlorination is the recommended solution to algae problems. For best results, adjust the pH to about 7.4, or even 7.2.

After superchlorinating, brush the walls vigorously, using a stainless-steel brush in concrete pools, or a soft nylon brush for vinyl-liner pools, then vacuum. Repeat the treatment if necessary to remove all algae spots. Pay particular attention to algae that forms around underwater light rims or where the ladder attaches to the pool. Keep the filter running continuously for 3 or 4 days and keep the chlorine residual to about 2.0 ppm. Don't allow swimming until the treatment is finished and the chlorine residual level has dropped to 3.0 or below. Remember, algae is easier to kill when immature. It gets progressively harder to remove the longer it has been allowed to grow.

Two of the most common and stubborn strains of algae are *black algae* and *yellow (mustard) algae.* Of the two, yellow algae is usually the easiest to brush off the walls, but will grow back quickly if not correctly treated. There is also a *green floating algae* that discolors the water. Superchlorination will handle this. Although chlorine is the first line of defense against algae growth, some strains appear to be almost chlorine resistant in stabilized pools and under favorable growth conditions. When this conditions develops, use of a commercial algaecide in addition to superchlorination and brushing is recommended. But if the instructions call for a quart of algaecide and you only use half a quart, nothing will have been accomplished. You must kill *all* algae or it will grow back at astonishing speed. Also, the filter circulation system must be kept running during treatment so that chlorine and the algaecide reach all parts of the pool and inside pipes and equipment.

Black algae grows in colonies and should be frequently brushed off pool walls during treatment. The reason is that the dead outside colonies protect the inner layers of algae from the chlorine or algaecide. To kill the entire colony, the dead layers must be brushed off. An effective algaecide will also provide some residual protection against algae reinfestation. And don't forget to thoroughly clean all brushes with a strong solution of bleach to kill any algae cells clinging to the fibers.

If algae has been allowed to grow and has gained too strong a foothold to be removed by treatment and brushing, it is recommended that you call in a pool service company. They will properly clean and sanitize the pool surfaces, in some cases using an acid-wash which is *strictly* the domain of trained professionals.

When the serviceman is there, ask how to prevent such severe cases of algae.

Stains

Plastered concrete pools can be stained by debris such as leaves, hairpins and other metal objects, algae, and mineral deposits. Metal objects should be removed from the pool immediately, to prevent rust stains from forming. On a plaster pool, you can buff away many stains with waterproof sandpaper. Pumice stones, available at pool supply stores, can also be used for scrubbing off hard-to-remove algae. You can either dive down to the area, or attach the stone to the end of your brush pole and work from above. Try to minimize damage to the plaster finish. Minute crevices and score marks make excellent breeding grounds for algae. *Do not* use pumice stones on tile. Strong detergent or chlorine will remove most stains from painted pools.

Scale

Scale is an accumulation of calcium carbonate. It can leave behind a stain when removed. As discussed earlier under "Water Balancing," such scale and staining will occur only when the water is out of balance. Scale can appear as a gray or brownish crust. Wet-or-dry sandpaper or an acid solution will remove fresh scale deposits, but if they have become established, then only *professional* acid-washing or power-sanding will usually remove them. them.

Stained or Corroded Fixtures

If fixtures are stained or corroded, the most probable cause is corrosively unbalanced water, often due to low pH. Bring the pH up to the recommended level (7.2 to 7.6). For additional insurance, bring up the level of calcium hardness as well.

Algae is easier to kill when immature. It gets progressively harder to remove the longer it has been allowed to grow.

The filter circulation system must be kept running during treatment so that chlorine and the algaecide reach all parts of the pool and inside pipes and equipment.

Eye Irritation and Chlorine Smells

Don't be fooled by this one. If skin and eye irritation occurs, or there is a distinct chlorine odor around the pool, the problem is too little chlorine, not too much. The solution is to superchlorinate the water to get rid of the chloramines. Adjust the pH to between 7.2 and 7.4 for maximum chlorine efficiency, then superchlorinate.

If You Have to Empty the Pool

There may be some water conditions so severe that you will have to empty the pool and start anew with fresh water. Always consult a pool service professional before undertaking such an ambitious procedure, and be sure to observe the precautions below.

Before emptying your pool, make sure the ground water table is below pool level. In early spring, for instance, the level of the water table can be higher than that of the pool water, due to spring runoff. The pressure exerted by ground water—called *hydrostatic pressure*—can severely damage the pool structure. Your local pool dealer should know about conditions in your area. Don't empty the pool if a storm is on its way or heavy rains are forecast.

Gather together all the chemicals, materials, and tools needed, so you can do the work quickly. If the pool is made of fiberglass, or is an above-ground pool, contact the builder to find out if, and how, the pool should be braced to prevent damage from water pressure in the ground or exerted by surrounding earth if it is empty. In areas where the water table is high, have a *hydrostatic relief valve* installed and make sure it is functioning during the wet season. Hydrostatic pressure can pop a concrete or fiberglass pool shell out of the ground when the pool is empty.

Water treatment is the foundation of pool maintenance. A pool with clean and properly balanced water will not only be free from bacteria and algae, but will also help to prevent mechanical failure that may result from untreated water. It may seem complicated, but you can easily develop a water treatment routine that won't be a burden in time or effort. It is important to emphasize that water treatment will only really be effective when it is properly and carefully done. That means all pool chemicals must be treated with extreme care. Read thoroughly, and follow exactly, all product and label directions. Store chemicals properly. The text on pages 84-85 gives everything you need to know about the safe handling of pool chemicals.

4 • Filtration Systems

The filtration system is the one essential piece of pool equipment. It is usually located close to the pump and heater. Water is pumped from the pool through pipes into the filter, then through the heater if there is one, before being returned to the pool. By circulating the water and filtering out large dirt particles and sediment that chemicals cannot handle, it enables you to use the same pool water over a long period of time. You need only add sufficient water to make up for evaporation, backwashing (cleaning the filter), and splash-out. But chemicals alone will not keep a pool sanitary and the water clean. An efficient filtration system does more than screen out dirt and debris—it also ensures the dispersion and mixture of sanitizing chemicals. This section describes the various types of filters, their operation and maintenance, and troubleshooting.

High-Rate Sand Filters

First introduced in the late 1950s, high-rate sand filters are popular and efficient. The basic system uses one deep, continuous layer of sand to filter dirt and debris particles out of the water (Figure 4.1). Trapped

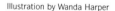
Illustration by Wanda Harper

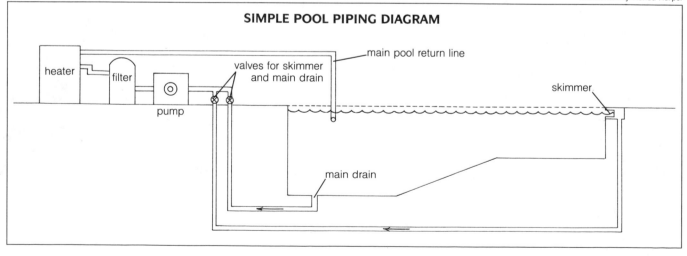

SIMPLE POOL PIPING DIAGRAM

heater

filter

pump

valves for skimmer and main drain

main pool return line

skimmer

main drain

WHAT COLOR IS YOUR SWIMMING POOL?

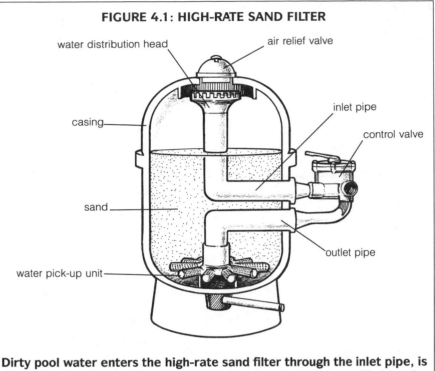

FIGURE 4.1: HIGH-RATE SAND FILTER

water distribution head

air relief valve

casing

inlet pipe

control valve

sand

outlet pipe

water pick-up unit

Dirty pool water enters the high-rate sand filter through the inlet pipe, is sprayed onto the sand by the distribution head, is then purified by the sand, and pumped back to the pool clean of dirt and debris.

> If your filter only has an inlet pressure gauge, it should be backwashed when the gauge shows an increase of 8 to 10 psi over the starting pressure — the pressure shown when the filter starts up after being cleaned.

dirt builds up in the sand until the water flow is greatly restricted, as well as the ability of the filter to do its job. There will be a resultant change in pressure on the pressure gauge, and this will indicate the need for backwashing. In the process of backwashing, the flow of water is reversed through the filter tank by turning the control valve to the backwash position. This creates an upward flow through the filter bed, which loosens dirt and dumps it into the wasteline.

High-rate filters require a particular type of sand. It is critical to use the correct size sand as recommended by the filter manufacturer. Sand just slightly larger or smaller than the specified particle size will render the filter less effective. The quantity of sand in the filter tank determines the amount of dirt the filter can hold. Put as much sand in the filter as possible, yet maintain a 10- to 12-inch *freeboard* (distance between the top of the sand bed and the lowest opening in the dis-

tributor). It is best, though, to check the recommendations of the filter manufacturer and follow them. A shallow sand bed will also work, but you will have to backwash more frequently.

At first, a high-rate sand filter with clean sand will remove only larger particles of dirt (between 12 to 15 microns in size). As the dirt builds up in the sand, the filter will remove finer and finer particles, eventually down to submicron size.

A typical high-rate sand filter is fitted with an inlet and outlet gauge. When the sand is clean, there will not usually be more than a 3 psi (pounds per square inch) differential between the two gauges. As the dirt builds up in the sand, the pressure on the inlet gauge will start to increase while the pressure shown on the outlet gauge will decrease. Most manufacturers recommend that when the pressure differential between the two gauges reaches 18 to 20 psi, the filter should be backwashed.

If your filter only has an inlet pressure gauge, it should be backwashed when the gauge shows an increase of 8 to 10 psi over the starting pressure — the pressure shown when the filter starts up after being cleaned. (The average starting pressure is 15 psi, but it should be stamped on the filter plate.) Backwashing too frequently doesn't allow the filter to do the maximum cleaning job necessary to achieve sparkling water, so you are not improving filtration by backwashing before the appropriate pressure difference registers on the gauge. Backwashing consists of reversing the flow of water from the top of the tank to the underdrain and switching the outlet water to the wasteline. Recommended backwashing time is about 2 to 3 minutes, or until the waste water runs clear. When the backwashing is finished, turn off the pump. This allows the sand bed to settle back and redistribute itself. Again, a filter-to-waste or rinse valve is often recommended, because if backwashing is not completely effective, a small amount of dirt will remain in the sand bed. When you start up the filter cycle again, a small puff of dirt will show up at the inlet opening in the pool. The filter-to-waste system diverts the first 20 seconds of flow to waste, which gets rid of the remaining dirt. The filtration system can then be returned to the full filter cycle.

Diatomaceous Earth Filters

The diatomaceous earth (DE) filter first appeared shortly after the end of the Second World War. Despite the introduction of high-rate sand filters, the DE filter is probably still the most widely used residential pool filter.

The DE filter gets its name from the filter media used – diatomaceous earth. Diatomaceous earth is a fine, chalky powder made from the fossilized remains of minute sea organisms (diatoms). Large deposits of diatomaceous earth have been found where ancient inland seas have dried up in areas such as California and Arizona. The deposits take the form of a soft rock formation, which is then mined. This soft rock is pulverized into a fine powder of talcumlike consistency. It is widely used as a filtering agent in breweries and dry cleaning plants as well.

There are various designs for DE filters, but basically the principle is the same. Within a tank, a series of filter grids are covered with a polypropylene or Dacron cloth (Figure 4.2). The most popular grid designs are curved, elliptical, flat plates (often called leaf-type DE filters), fingers, or round discs. The filter grids are kept in place by a manifold. In the center is a perforated tube. Water from the pool enters the tank, moves through the cloth grids and then back to the pool through the central tube. The filter is set into op-

eration, then a measured amount of diatomaceous earth is mixed with water into a slurry (a thin mixture of DE and water) and poured into the skimmer box, where it is sucked into the filter. The fine weave of the grid cloth is smaller than the individual particles of DE, so that the DE builds up a layer on the outside of the pad. This forms the actual filtering media. It is this DE media that does the filtering work, not the pads, and the DE layer must be thick enough to hold the dirt and keep it from reaching the pads. As this filter "cake" on the grids accumulates dirt and litter from the pool, it forms a resistance to the water flow. This shows as an increase in pressure on the filter gauge. When pressure reaches the manufacturer's stated level, the filter should be backwashed. On the backwash cycle, water flows up through the center inlet and forces the DE cake and accumulated dirt away from the cloth grids. The DE then falls off the grids and is flushed into the wasteline, and new DE is introduced into the filter.

There are two kinds of DE filters: the bag/pressure-type and the vacuum-type. The bag-type DE filter consists of a cloth bag inside the pressure tank. The bag is coated with DE, which filters the water before releasing it to the pool. This type of filter has to be opened to clean the expended DE from the bag before replacing it with new DE. Pressure-type filters have the filter pump connected to the inlet side from the pool.

Vacuum-type filters have the filter pump connected to the return side of the filter. Instead of pushing water through the filter, the pump sucks it through. In this manner, the filter unit works in conjunction with the skimmer, and a control filter normally allows you to draw water from the main pool drain or the vacuum outlet in the skimmer.

A new development in DE filters is the regeneration unit, which util-

When pressure reaches the manufacturer's stated level, the filter should be backwashed. On the backwash cycle, water flows up through the center inlet and forces the DE cake and accumulated dirt away from the cloth grids. The DE then falls off the grids and is flushed into the wasteline, and new DE is introduced into the filter.

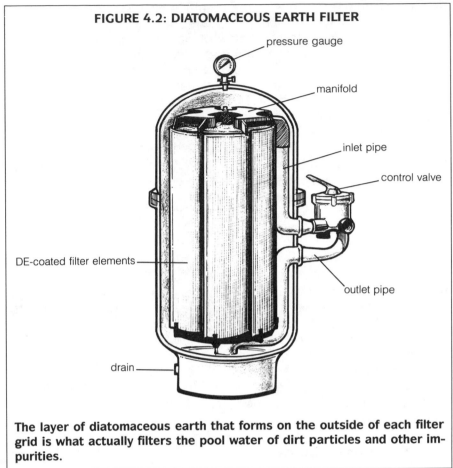

FIGURE 4.2: DIATOMACEOUS EARTH FILTER

pressure gauge

manifold

inlet pipe

control valve

DE-coated filter elements

outlet pipe

drain

The layer of diatomaceous earth that forms on the outside of each filter grid is what actually filters the pool water of dirt particles and other impurities.

izes flexible filter elements. As accumulated dirt clogs the DE cake around the elements, the filter rate slows down, as shown on the pressure gauge. A handle on the top of the filter allows regeneration of the filter without backwashing. Every 3 or 4 days, turn off the pump and move the handle down slowly and up sharply five or six times. Then switch the pump back on. What happens is that the handle shakes the clogged DE cake from the tubes so that it is remixed and then reapplied when the pump is switched on. Eventually the filter will need cleaning and a fresh supply of DE, but this is a simple procedure of switching off the pump and allowing the dirt and old DE to drain out.

There are two points to watch with all DE filters: one is not to add too much DE to the filter; the second is

not to add too little DE. Either too much or too little DE reduces filter efficiency. In disc- or leaf-type filters, too much DE can cause the DE cakes on the grids or discs to become so thick that they touch and compress against each other and then don't release during backwashing. Too little DE causes a more serious problem—it allows dirt to become embedded in and chafe the cloth grids, which can ruin them. Grid replacement is costly.

Occasionally it may be necessary to remove and wash the cloth grids to clean away body oils and any embedded dirt. Calcium may also adhere to the cloth and clog it. One common method is to wash each the grids in a 25 percent solution of muriatic acid (one part acid to four parts water). Rinse thoroughly with water, then wash each grid with a mild household soap solution. Rinse again to remove any soap film. Before reassembly, closely inspect the grids and repair any small holes with fingernail polish or silicon sealer. Grids that are too damaged to be repaired this way must be replaced. Don't forget to check out the interior of the tank before replacing the filter grids, and remove any debris before reinstalling them. Remember how fine DE is—the smallest hole in the pads or valve components will allow it to escape into the pool.

In many areas of the country, you cannot backwash DE filters into the city or town sewer system. In this case, a separation tank is included with the filter. Smaller than the filter, it contains a fine mesh bag that collects the DE during the backwash cycle. Make sure entrapped air has been bled from the separation tank and filter system before backwashing. The bag can then be removed from the tank and emptied elsewhere.

Cartridge Filters

Cartridge filters are relatively new components for the in-ground pool, becoming available only in the last decade (Figure 4.3). For a number of years, cartridge filters of resin-impregnated cardboard or a foam-type cartridge filter have been used for small in-ground or above-ground pool systems, but only recently has the technology been developed to make them suitable for larger in-ground, residential pools. As with sand or DE filters, there is a filter tank that holds one or several cartridges, similar to the filter found in a car air cleaner. The *septum* (filtering medium) consists of a special filter paper or polyester cloth, supported at each end by caps. It is usually pleated to provide maximum filtering surface area. The main difference is that cartridge filters cannot be backwashed. They must be removed from the tank and washed by hand. You can use a garden hose

with a high-pressure nozzle to do this. The main advantage of this type of filter is its simplicity. It also conserves the heated and chemically treated water which is normally lost through backwashing systems. Large-size cartridge and multiple cartridge filters are now available to extend the time between cleaning cycles.

The life expectancy of a cartridge can be anywhere from 1 and 8 years, depending on the quality of the element and the care given it. A pressure gauge shows when the cartridge needs cleaning (follow manufacturer's instructions). As dirt builds up, it slows down the flow of water and increases the pressure. To clean the cartridge, switch off the pump and remove the cartridge. Hose it down, using a high-pressure

Cartridge filters cannot be backwashed.

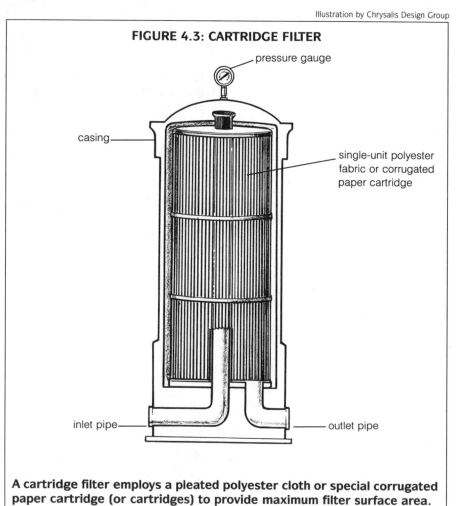

FIGURE 4.3: CARTRIDGE FILTER

pressure gauge

casing

single-unit polyester fabric or corrugated paper cartridge

inlet pipe

outlet pipe

A cartridge filter employs a pleated polyester cloth or special corrugated paper cartridge (or cartridges) to provide maximum filter surface area.

WHAT COLOR IS YOUR SWIMMING POOL?

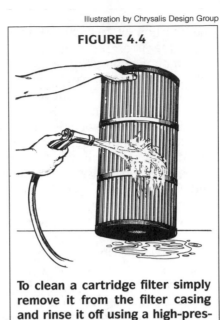

FIGURE 4.4

To clean a cartridge filter simply remove it from the filter casing and rinse it off using a high-pressure hose nozzle.

If possible, ask to have a bypass valve installed between the pump and cartridge filter so that you can vacuum directly into the wasteline without running dirt and debris through the cartridge.

hose nozzle (Figure 4.4). Pay particular attention to dirt that becomes jammed between the flutes or pleats of the cartridge. There are cartridge cleaners available to help soak off embedded dirt. If you don't do a thorough job of cleaning, the cartridge will become so clogged that not only will the filter cycle work less efficiently, but it will ruin the cartridge. Replace the cartridge or cartridges when they are obviously worn and/or fail to do the job necessary to clean the water.

If possible, ask to have a bypass valve installed between the pump and cartridge filter so that you can run the vacuum directly into the wasteline without putting it through the cartridge. A heavy dirt load vacuumed through the cartridge filter will badly clog it, and sometimes the sudden heavy load may even destroy the cartridge.

Body oils, suntan lotions and creams can all reduce the efficiency of the filter system, no matter what kind of system you employ. The use of a hot water spa connected to the pool greatly increases the problem of body oil contamination from perspiration. These oils form a film over the filter media, producing a false

clogging or caking. Ask swimmers to shower with soap and water first, and try to minimize the use of suntan lotions and creams by people swimming in the pool. If they are used, try to encourage the application of biodegradable sun products. Commercial cartridge-cleaning solutions (available at pool supply stores) can be used to soak away the oil film.

IMPORTANT FILTER COMPONENTS

Although pool filters can be complex, computerized, and mystifying, it is not unrealistic for pool owners to keep the system running smoothly simply by understanding the components which are not only crucial to its operation, but the source of many problems. If you have knowledge of basic filter operation, and learn how to recognize trouble when it is still easy to fix, then you'll be in good shape. The text below is an introduction to pool filters, considerations, and components, and is the place from which you should be able to maintain the system for years to come.

Filter Valves

Valves and fittings play an important part in the filtration system. They regulate and direct the flow of water through the pool and filtration system. Leaking or worn valves should be detected and professionally repaired or replaced as soon as possible, before they can cause damage to the system.

There are a number of different types of valves, but the most common are rotary valves, ball valves, and multiport valves. Ask what kind of valves your system employs and familiarize yourself with the look and operation of the filter and its valve components. In the event that anything goes wrong, you may be in a position to help the repairman locate and fix the problem. Below is a brief description of the three most commonly used valves in pool filter systems.

Rotary valves were among the second generation of valves developed for pool filters and are not much used in new pool systems. They employ a tube-type body, in which the water direction is changed by a set of plates and O-rings within the tube. This enabled extra positions to be added, which then allowed water to bypass the filter, return to the pool, as well as have it pumped into the wasteline without first going through the filter.

Ball valves allow control over the force and direction of water (Figure 4.5). They are available as two-way, three-way, and four-way valves. They use Teflon seats and neoprene O-rings for tight sealing, and are easy to replace by unscrewing the assembly nut.

The most commonly used valve in filter systems today is the *multiport valve*. This valve contains a moveable port which can be rotated to select up to six functions, usually shown on top of the valve, such as backwash, filter, rinse, waste, and closed (Figure 4.6). DO NOT change the function of a multiport valve while the filter pump is running. Switch off the pump first. If not, the rubber segmented gasket in this type of valve can be destroyed.

If you have reason to believe that the filter valves are impairing performance of the system because of dirt and debris, corrosion, wear, or improper assembly, inspect the filter and its valve components for these adverse conditions to the extent that you are able. *Do not* even attempt to disassemble the filter if you are at all unsure about how to do it. In any case, valve repair and replacement is work that requires professional experience. Call in a service company and share with the repairman your observations at the source of the problem.

Skimmer Boxes

Automatic skimmer boxes operate when the filter is on and provide a vital link in the filtration system by removing debris that falls into the water. The skimmer is built into the side of the pool during construction, and some pools are fitted with several skimmers. Most skimmers today are made from a high-density,

DO NOT change the function of a multi-port valve while the filter pump is running.

Illustration by Chrysalis Design Group

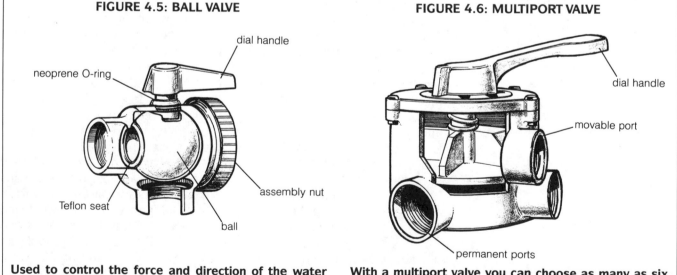

FIGURE 4.5: BALL VALVE

dial handle

neoprene O-ring

Teflon seat

ball

assembly nut

Used to control the force and direction of the water through the filter, ball valves offer two, three, and four flow variations.

FIGURE 4.6: MULTIPORT VALVE

dial handle

movable port

permanent ports

With a multiport valve you can choose as many as six different valve functions (such as backwash, filter, waste, closed) simply by engaging a single movable part.

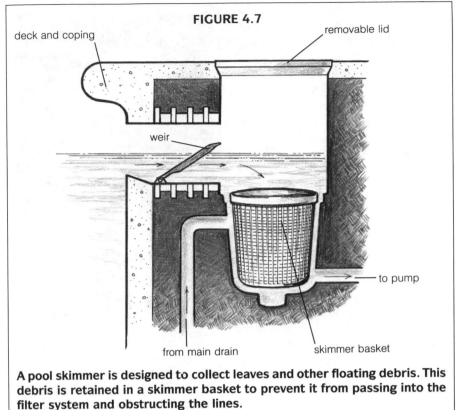

FIGURE 4.7

deck and coping

removable lid

weir

to pump

from main drain

skimmer basket

A pool skimmer is designed to collect leaves and other floating debris. This debris is retained in a skimmer basket to prevent it from passing into the filter system and obstructing the lines.

> The skimmer opening faces the pool, with a *weir* flap or hinge at the front of the opening.

noncorrosive plastic (Figure 4.7). The molded shell is recessed into the pool wall at the waterline, with a drain and a suction line fitting molded into the shell. The skimmer opening faces the pool, with a *weir* flap or hinge at the front of the opening. It is this weir or gate that creates the skimming action—clearing off dirt, algae, leaves, and other floating rubbish from the surface of the pool before it has a chance to settle to the bottom. The debris is then trapped in the strainer basket (Figure 4.8).

The strainer basket of the skimmer box should be cleaned daily under normal conditions and more frequently when leaves are falling or high winds are blowing large amounts of litter into the pool. A clogged strainer can restrict the flow of water to the filter pump to such an extent that the pump can stall and damage the motor. If, for some reason, you have a pool without a built-in, automatic skimmer, you can

buy a vacuum-type skimmer that floats on the surface of the pool and connects to the pool vacuum line.

The weir flap in the throat of the built-in skimmer is the critical piece of the system. The weir is used to direct surface water only into the skimmer. Water flows into the skimmer (drawn by the filter pump) at a rate of about 1¼ gallons per second. Without the weir, the speed or velocity of the water is too slow to efficiently draw debris into the skimmer. But with the weir in place, the pump draws water faster over the top of the weir at a depth of only about three-sixteenths of an inch. With this fast movement of surface water comes efficient skimming of the pool surface. This results in less running time for the filter and less chance that leaves and other debris will sink to the bottom of the pool.

Most skimmers incorporate a fitting to allow the attachment of a hose for vacuuming the pool. The vacuum hose fits over the opening into the skimmer strainer basket. Some models even incorporate a cartridge filter below the skimmer basket for additional protection of the pump and filter units. There are skimmer models available with automatic chlorine dispensers and low-water protection devices that shut off the pump or add water to the pool automatically when the water level drops below the skimmer opening. This prevents air from entering the filter pipes, pump, and filter which can cause malfunction.

The automatic skimmer is usually set to handle about half of all the water going from the pool to the filter. The other half is usually drawn through other pool drains. When vacuuming, make sure the valves controlling the water flow from the main drain and skimmer are reset correctly. The line from the main drain to the filter has to be closed off when you vacuum to ensure a strong suction action from the filter pump. When vacuuming has been completed, make sure the main drain line has been reopened about halfway and the skimmer line has been similarly adjusted. If the skimmer line is closed off too much, no skimming action will take place.

There is little that can go wrong with a skimmer. The main problems

Photograph courtesy of Baker Hydro, Inc.

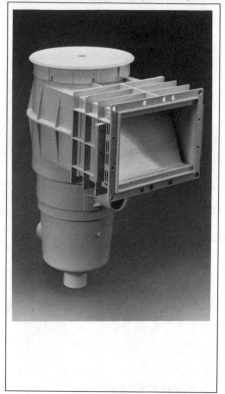

Illustration by Chrysalis Design Group

FIGURE 4.8

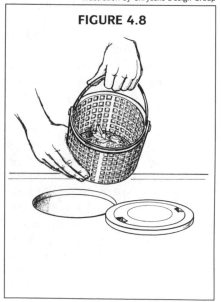

encountered are usually the result of the basket becoming jammed with leaves and debris, or the weir flap getting knocked out of place. There is a thick buoyant piece across the top of the weir to ensure that it floats high in the water. Because of its buoyancy the weir flap is susceptible to all kinds of trouble: it can be bent out of shape, broken, become unattached, or even "disappear." These problems are easy to correct. A not-so-easy problem to fix is when the skimmer basket is damaged or when the pipe to the filter becomes blocked because of careless cleaning of the skimmer basket. Turn off the power, and if you're lucky, you may be able to fish out the obstruction. If not, you may have to use a plumber's snake or disconnect the pipe at the filter pump and try to force the obstruction back out with water pressure from a hose. A pool plumbing expert is your last resort, but if the pipe is really jammed, it is advisable to get his help rather than try to relieve the blockage yourself.

The strainer basket of the skimmer box should be cleaned daily under normal conditions and more frequently when leaves are falling or high winds are blowing large amounts of litter into the pool.

WHAT COLOR IS YOUR SWIMMING POOL?

Filter Sizing

No matter what kind of filter you choose for your pool, either as a new installation or replacement, the most important factor to remember is that the filter system must be sized to the volume of water in the pool. It is far better to slightly over-size the filter and pump, than to use a filter that is too small for the pool. A pump that is too small for the filter may not backwash adequately. The recommended turnover time for a pool (the time it takes for the filter system to filter the entire body of water) is about 8 hours. This does not necessarily mean the filter must run this number of hours daily to ensure clean water. In fact, with correctly balanced water that has the recommended levels of free or available sanitizer, some pool owners have found that they can reduce filtration to 6, 4, and sometimes as little as 2 hours daily. But short filter cycles must be developed to conform to individual pool conditions and requirements, which may vary from season to season. It used to be that filters were turned on for 8 or 12 hours a day (sometimes more), but the high cost of electricity has led the pool industry to investigate how many hours of filtration are actually needed each day. It turned out to be much less time than anyone thought.

Nevertheless, the filter system should be sized to the pool. This means that the pump (motor) and filter must all be sized to each other. The basic rule is to size the pump and motor to the pool capacity, then size the filter (its flow rate and capacity) to the pump. A competent pool equipment dealer or pool builder will be happy to work this out for you when you provide him with all the relevant information. With good advice, you should be able to make an appropriate choice. But remember if the filter is too small, it won't keep the pool clean. And if the filter is too large, it will cost you

The basic rule is to size the pump and motor to the pool capacity, then size the filter (its flow rate and capacity) to the pump.

The formation of mud balls in the sand generally results from seriously imbalanced water or insufficient backwashing.

more to buy, but not necessarily more to operate. Don't opt for the minimum size filter to fit your requirements. Such a filter may work fine under normal conditions, but any sudden influx of dirt and debris from heavy rain and wind could quickly overload the filter.

With the readiness of reputable pool equipment dealers to supply you with the right components, I would suggest that you get the recommendations of several reliable pool dealers and filter manufacturers before you update or replace the filtration system. Many dealers offer free estimates. With these in hand, you can make your selection based on price and filter preference.

TROUBLESHOOTING FOR FILTERS

Pool water that has been well maintained should make your filter system practically trouble free. There are a few conditions, especially in the older sand filters, that may require your attention. Otherwise, filter care is pretty elementary.

Sand Filters

One of the main advantages of sand filters is their reliability—they require minimal maintenance. Air leakage in the tank or the accumulation of mud balls in the sand, which causes a condition known as channeling, are about the only problems one normally encounters.

Mud balls. The formation of mud balls in the sand generally results from seriously imbalanced water or insufficient backwashing. Water with a high pH cannot hold a great amount of calcium in solution; it precipitates the excess calcium so that it accumulates on the floor of the pool. The calcium is sucked up during vacuuming and is deposited in the filter sand. Such calcification can also cause scale to form inside the filter valve, reducing efficiency and

Illustration by Wanda Harper

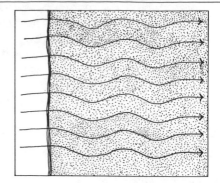

1. Filter sand is clean and pool water flows easily through it.

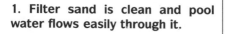
mud balls

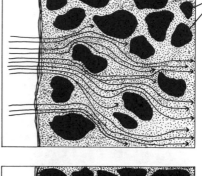

2. Mud balls form when pool water is unbalanced and impede the filtering process.

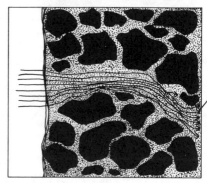
channeling

3. Channeling occurs when the water is so unbalanced and the filter media so dirty that pool water passes unfiltered through a system of channels created by huge mud balls.

eventually causing a bypass condition to occur, which can render the filter virtually useless. If calcification has been occurring in your pool for some time, it would be advisable to have this condition treated by your pool serviceman.

One indication of mud balls is that the filter needs backwashing more frequently. The only way to find out if mud balls are the problem is to open the filter and check the sand bed. In the most serious cases, you'll notice **channeling**, a condition that will be obvious. There will be an open passage or channel down one side or segment of the filter so that water just passes down

the channel into the collector and back to the pool without filtration. This does not happen all at once. There are several stages before channeling occurs.

As stated before, calcium collects in the filter and adheres to the sand grains. It is not removed by backwashing. Gradually, the sand grains join together and accumulate hair and lint to form mud balls. As the mud balls get larger, they join together to form larger mud balls, which eventually block one part of the filter, forcing the water to travel through only a small segment of sand. The large mud block, which can occupy one-half to two-thirds of

> One indication of mud balls is that the filter needs backwashing more frequently.

WHAT COLOR IS YOUR SWIMMING POOL?

Relieve *all* trapped air prior to working on a filter or pump.

The most obvious cause of an air leak is that the water level in the pool has been allowed to get so low that air is being drawn in through the skimmer.

the filter media, also forces water up this channel during backwashing, piling loose sand on top of it. If, on inspection of the sand, you find about 20 percent of the sand media blocked with mud balls, the best course is to dump it and replace with new sand.

If there is only a small number of mud balls, you can dissolve them. Turn off the filter pump and drain as much water as possible from the filter tank. Then pour in a solution of one part muriatic acid to one part water. Add the acid to the water in a plastic bucket. You could also buy a commercial filter cleaner. Leave this solution in the filter for about 4 to 6 hours, then backwash thoroughly. This treatment should break down most of the calcification and dissolve the mud balls.

If the sand has to be replaced, also check the collector tube openings in the bottom of the filter. These are very small and scale or debris can block them. Most commercial filter cleaners will remove scale, but other types of blockage may require mechanical removal. Make sure the openings are free and clear, but do **not** use a steel probe—this could enlarge the openings. Use a small-bristled brush or a plastic probe instead.

Air leaks. The second problem involves air in the filter tank. It is important to mention that trapped air in the filter system can be dangerous. Relieve *all* trapped air prior to working on a filter or pump. Over a period of time, air will become locked in the lines simply through its normal operation. If your filter has a manual air bleed system, you should release the air once a week to avoid pressure from air buildup. And if you are going to disassemble the filter or the pump, *always* bleed the air before you begin work. Most new filters feature an automatic air bleed system, but if yours is an older model, do take care to relieve air pressure before you begin repairs of any kind.

Most air problems involve leaks at some point in the filtration system. Leaks on the suction side of the pump should be suspected if there are excessive air bubbles entering the pool from the return line, or if there is air blowing back through the main drain or surface skimmer when the filter is turned off. Sometimes an air leak will cause the gauges to vibrate or not register any pressure at all. If the air leak is on the discharge side of the filter pump, you can often hear a bubbling sound in the filter tank each time the filter is turned off.

Finding the air leak involves a process of elimination. The most obvious cause is that the water level in the pool has been allowed to get so low that air is being drawn in through the skimmer. Check the level and adjust, if necessary. The next most obvious place to check is the pump's leaf strainer. If the gasket is worn or the lid is not tightened sufficiently on the leaf strainer, air can be sucked in. Your local pool supply store should have a replacement lid or gasket, and while you're there ask to be sure that you know exactly how to install the new component.

More troublesome to detect and correct is a leak from the front of the impeller on the pump. If this is the case, see the troubleshooting section on pumps and motors (pages 39-43). The packing or seals on valves and other fittings can become worn or loose which can cause leaks. But before trying to inspect these components, make sure that the large O-ring which seals together the two halves of the filter tank is not worn, dry, or incorrectly seated. If dry, the ring should be lubricated with a special silicone O-ring grease, available from pool service companies—do not use petroleum jelly. If cracked or misshapen, it must be replaced. If you decide to replace the O-ring yourself get instructions or directions from your owner's manual or a pool service company, and then thoroughly clean the new O-ring and tank before reassembly. If you cannot find the source of the air leak or care not to attempt repair on your own, it may be best to call in an expert from the manufacturer, distributor, or pool service company. Whatever you finally decide to do, don't tear down the fittings or pump and then expect a professional to reassemble it without a fee. The work is not extremely difficult, but it does require a certain amount of mechanical aptitude.

Filter Preventive Maintenance

To keep all filter systems operating without trouble or incident, follow these basic rules.

- Keep the filter media clean at all times.
- Repair any air leaks at the piping connection or filter gaskets.
- Have gaskets replaced when they become nicked, gouged, inoperative, or otherwise worn.
- Oil all moving parts at the loca-

tions specified by a pool service professional or the owner's manual.
- Remove dirt, leaves, hair, and other debris from the pump leaf strainer regularly.

For more technical information on filter assembly, operation, and maintenance, consult the materials that were provided by the manufacturer with the filter. Or ask your pool service company or store if they can recommend reading materials.

Without a filter in good working condition your pool will become both dirty and unhealthy in a matter of days. Maintaining the filtration system is often a matter of common sense: establishing and following a maintenance routine, cleaning or backwashing filter components, emptying out the leaf strainer or skimmer box basket, and being attentive to strange sounds or indications will serve as a good foundation for filter care. But in the event of filter complications that are beyond your capacity to remedy, call in a pool serviceman.

5 • Pumps and Motors

Because pumps and motors are invariably sold as an integral unit, this discussion will treat them that way, and refer to the combined unit as the pump. Pump motors are electrically powered and need little or no maintenance. Most are sealed units that do not require lubrication, but some may require periodic oiling. The motor and pump unit are connected by an airtight, watertight seal and are normally mounted on a single frame. It is this combination of motor and pump that draws water from the pool, forces it through the filter, and sends it back to the pool. Most filter systems sold today come with pump and motor included as part of the filter package.

SIZING A PUMP

The size of the pump is not a hit-or-miss thing. A pump that is too powerful for the system can damage the filter. If the pump is too small, the filter won't work correctly and

Photo courtesy of Sta-Rite Industries, Inc.

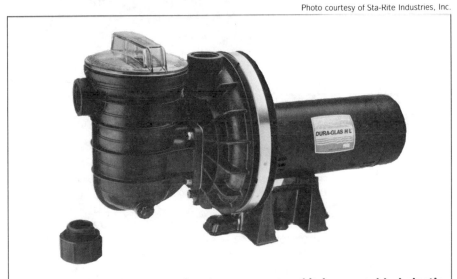

Most modern pool pumps and motors are encased in heavy molded plastic to prevent wear from exposure to the elements and corrosion.

neither will other accessories such as the skimmer, vacuum attachment, or the automatic vacuuming unit.

The recommended sequence of events is to size the pump capacity to the pool gallonage and desired turnover rate, then size the filter to the pump. When it comes to the filter, always err on the big side. You can choose a filter that has a larger capacity than your needs without any problem, but if the filter is too small for the pump then you could get yourself in trouble. Read the literature provided by manufacturers, do a little math, and ask intelligent questions of your pool builder or service company. In this way, you will get a system that accommodates both your needs and that of the pool.

To size a pump you need to take into account not only the pool gallonage and turnover rate, but also back pressure (also termed head loss or hydraulic head), horsepower needed, the length in feet of straight pipe, and the number of elbows and fittings in the system. For the uninitiated, these factors can make the process of calculation difficult. That's why it is customarily the job of the pool builder to properly size the pump and circulation system for maximum efficiency or, in the case of an older pool being updated, the job of the pool service company or contractor.

MOTOR DESIGN AND COMPONENTS

Electric motors for pumps are available in a wide range of sizes (horsepower), with different starter systems and casing materials. But basically, electric motors follow the same mechanical principles. A large number of copper wire coils are wound and woven together to form windings (called field coils) which take up most of the space inside the cylindrical casing of the motor.

Through the hollow center of these windings is a shaft, held in place by bearings at each end of the motor. This shaft carries the armature—an iron and copper electromagnet, which is free to revolve inside the hollow center of the windings. When the motor is switched on an electric current (either 110 or 220 volts) passes through the windings and creates a strong electromagnetic force that turns the armature and shaft at a high speed. The high speed revolutions of the shaft drive the pump.

Starting the motor, however, is like starting your car—it requires much more energy to start the motor than it does to run it at full speed. To provide this extra shove of electricity, motors have a starting switch mechanism. Two switch types are commonly used: *centrifugal*, which provides an extra boost of electricity when operation of the motor begins; and *capacitor*, which stores enough of an electric current in a capacitor to start the motor.

The windings, armature, starter switch, and other motor components are enclosed inside a casing of metal or high-density plastic. There are two main types of casing—drip-proof and completely enclosed. Both types of casing work well if correctly sited and cared for.

The *drip-proof casing* has partially open ends for ventilation. A small fan is connected to the front shaft inside the casing, to draw in air through entry holes. The air is blown back through the windings and armature, cooling them, and out through the back of the pump. With this type of casing, moisture and dust can foul the starter windings and the small gap between the armature and windings. Water spilled or sprayed onto the motor can short-circuit it. Overheating can occur on hot days, particularly if the motor is poorly ventilated and the pump is working hard. Most modern motors feature a thermal overload switch that turns off the motor at a

> The recommended sequence of events is to size the pump capacity to the pool gallonage and desired turnover rate, then size the filter to the pump. When it comes to the filter, always err on the big side.

preset temperature or maximum current draw. This gives the motor a chance to cool down. It can be restarted by pushing the reset switch, but wait until the motor has cooled down.

The *completely enclosed casing* has a fan mounted at the back of the motor, which is enclosed in a small shield, rather than inside the casing as with the drip-proof type. This casing prevents water, dampness or dust from entering the motor and switch gears. This does not mean you can freely allow water and litter to gather around the motor. Some water could seep inside and cause a short-circuit, but this type of casing is most appropriate for pool conditions because it provides the best protection for the pump and motor.

Pool motors and pumps should be installed in a cool, clean, dry location so that dust, leaves, and other debris won't clog the motor's ventilation passages. Don't install a pool motor and pump anywhere near the laundry room. Lint from dryers will be sucked up by the motor fan and clog the air intake. The motor should be covered and slightly elevated so that water puddles will not be sucked into the motor by the cooling fan. Ideally, the motor and pump unit should be enclosed in a waterproof structure with louvered sides to provide ventilation and protection

from rain. Some manufacturers will not guarantee motors unless they have been protected in this way.

Most pump motors are single speed, but dual speed motors are available. There is considerable difference of opinion within the pool industry about these two-speed motors. The main shortcoming of the two-speed pump is that if not carefully sized to the filter and the pool, it sometimes doesn't pump enough water when running on the lower speed. The advantage is that it can save energy. The original two-speed motor/pump was run on low speed at night and high or normal speed during the day. Some modern two-speed pumps use high speed to overcome initial back pressure in the system, then drop to the lower speed for energy savings. Available now are energy efficient single-speed pumps. Set to run the specified number of hours with a time clock, significant energy savings can be realized. Time clocks are simple 24-hour timing mechanisms that turn the motor on and off at specified times, night or day.

Most modern swimming pool pumps are self-priming, which means that the pump is always full of water and does not need to be primed with water before starting. Many pumps still found on older pools are "regular" pumps (not self-priming). If such a pump loses its

Illustration by Wanda Harper

A motor cover will provide essential protection and proper ventilation for the motor and its components.

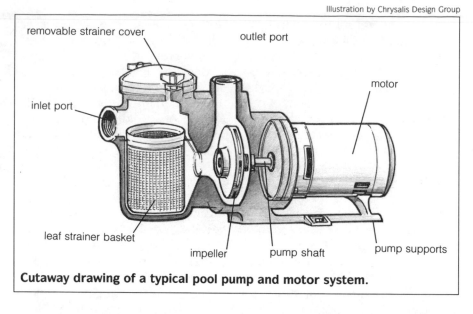

removable strainer cover

outlet port

motor

inlet port

leaf strainer basket

impeller

pump shaft

pump supports

Cutaway drawing of a typical pool pump and motor system.

priming charge, the motor can overheat during operation, damaging both the motor and pump.

A *leaf strainer* is a standard feature of most pump units sold today. It catches leaves, hair, lint, and other large particles of debris before they can enter and clog the pump. It also holds a reservoir of water to self-prime the pump. Many strainers have a clear, see-through plastic top so you don't have to remove it to see if the basket needs emptying. The strainer should be cleaned regularly. When clogged, it will greatly reduce the flow of water to the filter.

The pump body or volute holds the components of the pump, including the *impeller*, which actually pumps the water. Two basic types are used—open vane and shrouded vane. When the impeller spins, water or air is thrown out from the center by the vanes on the impeller, which lowers pressure there and creates the pumping action.

In some cases, the impeller works in conjunction with a *diffuser*. The diffuser is a round, flat plate which also has raised radiating fins. It faces the impeller with a narrow gap between the two sets of fins or vanes. Over a period of time, this diffuser plate can be gouged or worn by tiny bits of gravel or sand that pass through the strainer. Some pumps feature a

stainless steel wear plate to reduce damage to the diffuser. How much water a pump can move is determined by the depth of the vanes on the impeller. If you install an impeller with deeper vanes, you must also increase the horsepower of the pump.

One other critical component of the pump is the mechanical seal that stops water from leaking out around the shaft between the pump and electric motor. These mechanical seals are commonly a spring-loaded, rubber-cased unit, which are routinely replaced whenever the

The diffuser is a round, flat plate which also has raised radiating fins.

vane

direction
of rotation

The pump's impeller has raised vanes that circulate the pool water and actually move it through the system.

WHAT COLOR IS YOUR SWIMMING POOL?

> When starting a pump
> after repair work, or if the
> pump has been off for
> some time, always make
> sure there is water in it.

pump is professionally disassembled for other repairs. Both types utilize ceramic and carbon parts.

The ceramic and carbon seals are delicate and can be easily cracked if tapped with a screwdriver or other metal object. It is good to know where the seal is and how to identify damage to it. If you determine that it needs to be replaced, call in a pool serviceman and observe him as he works on the seal. It is really the job of a professional to disassemble a pump and replace worn or damaged seals.

When starting a pump after repair work, or if the pump has been off for some time, always make sure there is water in it. With a self-priming pump, make sure the strainer pot is full of water. Open all suction and discharge valves that may have been closed and bleed the air from the filter tank before trying to start the pump.

TROUBLESHOOTING FOR PUMPS AND MOTORS

If you asked manufacturers of pump systems about the most frequent problems encountered by their service people in the field, you'll find the answers revealing. Keep in mind that the relationship between the pump and motor is a close one—defects in the pump can affect the motor and vice versa. On the pages that follow you will find typical service problems, how to detect them, and how (if it is reasonable) to repair the trouble.

Malfunction may occur for the following reasons: lack of lubrication in the moving parts; overtightening of fittings; incorrectly set valves; faulty hose installation allowing air to be drawn into the pump; incorrect sizing of pump to filter; incorrect sizing of pipe to head loss (back-pressure); incorrect plumbing with too many elbows and other restrictions; incorrect electrical wiring; wrong voltage supply to pump; debris in the pump strainer and impeller housing; sizing pump by horsepower instead of by pump performance curve; poor protection from roof water runoff and accumulated water beneath motor; and undersized pipes on suction side of pump.

It is simply not practical to try to cover everything that can go wrong with a motor or pump—this book isn't meant to be a repair manual for one thing. For another, the variables of installation, environmental conditions, maintenance, use, the particulars of each pump and motor, and human error make it a difficult task. Instead, I will try to cover the most common problems that apply to pumps and motors in a general way.

Be careful. Never work on **any** electrical equipment such as motors and pumps without first disconnecting the power supply. The information given in this book on filters, pumps, and motors is meant to provide greater understanding. It is not a recommendation to do this work yourself, nor does it presume to be the last word on diagnosis and repair. You should always consult the manufacturer's literature first and follow the recommendations given if you feel capable. Pay particular attention to any provisions that would void the warranty if the work is not done by a qualified technician. If you have any questions or concerns about the operation or repair of the pump, motor, or filter, it is advisable to consult a reputable pool maintenance contractor before you attempt any work. It is always best to call in a qualified repairman to perform all but the most elementary repairs.

Motor doesn't run. You switch on the pump motor and nothing happens: what do you do? Go through a process of elimination, starting with the obvious:

1. The power is turned off at the main supply—check it.

2. The circuit breaker is out or the fuse blown. If the reset breaker or replaced fuse fails again, the problem is a serious overload on the circuit, probably caused by a short-circuit in the motor itself.

Presumably, these are the reasons a motor won't start. But it may also be the time clock. It may be set to start the pump at 2 p.m. and you're trying to start it at noon. Reset the timer or switch it to the manual (OFF) position. If the motor still won't start, check to be sure that the main power supply is turned on, then check the circuit breaker or fuse. If these are okay, turn off the power to the motor and check to see if the casing is abnormally hot. If so, chances are the thermal overload switch has been activated. Most pool pumps have an automatic overload switch, which will reactivate the pump when the motor cools down. Older pumps may have a manual reset button. If the motor now runs without further problems, fine. But beware that something caused the motor to overheat. It could be that the motor is undersized for the load, moisture could have gotten inside the pump, or perhaps there is a temporary blockage in the intake line from the pool. Make it a habit to check the intake lines to the pool before starting the pump and motor. The skimmer basket may be jammed with debris or leaves, or something else could be blocking the main drain.

Assuming that the pump has not overheated and the time clock is not shutting off power, check the main power supply switch and circuit breaker or fuse. Most local regulations require a separate circuit for the motor/pump system, that is, there are no other outlets on that line. If the power line is not separate, and the fuse has burned or the breaker popped out, chances are the line has been overloaded, probably by trying to start the pump while some other equipment is also drawing power on that line. If so, have a pool electrician wire a separate circuit for the pool equipment at the earliest opportunity. Turn off any other appliances on that line before restarting the pump. If the circuit breaker pops again or the fuse blows, there is a short somewhere, and that will have to be located and corrected. Call in a licensed electrician or a pool equipment repairman to have the pump/motor unit tested for short-circuits and restored to working order.

If the pump is not overly hot to the touch, the power supply is turned on, the circuit breaker or fuse is okay, the reset button has been activated, and the time clock is on manual—and the motor still won't start—what next? Look carefully at the wiring for a loose connection. Don't attempt to correct any wiring defect without first turning off the power. The next thing to check is the switch itself. Again, not without first turning off the power. The most common problem on a centrifugal motor is that the centrifugal switch spring has broken. This must be replaced. On a capacitor motor, it is the capacitor that has probably shorted out.

Motor runs but is noisy. If the motor makes a humming sound, there are a number of possibilities: bearings are worn and are beginning to seize, the centrifugal switch spring has failed, or there is a burned out starter winding. Noise can be the result of rust, lack of lubrication, or improper wear. Try as best you can to locate the source of the noise and the problem, and then get the advice of a pool serviceman.

Motor bearings. The bearings at either end of the armature shaft in the pump motor are usually the sealed-type. In this kind of bearing the lubricant is sealed inside the bearing so it cannot be lubricated from outside as with the older kind of bearings. With proper care, such

Don't attempt to correct any wiring defect without first turning off the power.

bearings will last a long time, but age and overload causes them to wear. Over a period of time, the sealed lubricant is used up. When this happens, the bearings start to rattle. That is the time to put in new bearings—don't wait until they begin to whine. From a whine, they will progress to a scream, which means the bearings are not only dry inside, but are wearing down at a high rate of speed. This causes the shaft to spin off center from its exact central axis. When this happens, the armature can touch the windings, shorting out the motor. And repairing or replacing the motor windings is far more expensive than installing new bearings. Some bearings are fitted with a plastic collar. If the motor is allowed to run with noisy bearings, they will eventually seize, melting the collar, and the only answer will be a new motor. Don't ignore bearing problems: make an appointment to have them repaired or replaced as soon as you suspect trouble.

Pump won't run. If the pump doesn't operate, the first things to check are the inlet and outlet valves—are they open or has someone accidentally closed them? Is the water level in the pool so low that the inlet in the skimmer cannot draw in water? If so, correct the water level. Check the skimmer box and clean it out if plugged with leaves and debris. Perhaps the weir flap has jammed, preventing water from flowing into the skimmer? Next, check the leaf strainer on the pump. Empty the basket, if necessary, and make sure the strainer pot is full of water before replacing the lid. Be sure that the strainer pot isn't cracked or leaking—if so, it will have to be repaired or replaced. Look at the flexible couplings and plastic fittings on the pump to ensure they are not cracked or leaking.

The same checks apply to an above-ground pool, with some exceptions. If the pump does not have a leaf strainer, debris may have bypassed the skimmer and jammed or fouled the impeller, or the impeller may have shattered inside the pump. If the pool has an "over-the-wall" type skimmer, make sure all the air has been removed from the line.

Pump is not operating properly. If the pump has been working fine but suddenly stops, is greatly reduced in flow, or is making strange noises, check for the following: a blockage in the suction line; a valve closed on the outlet; the backwash valve is in the wrong position; new filter medium (on DE and cartridge filters) may have been replaced incorrectly; the impeller is broken; a nonreturn valve (typically placed between heater and filter) may have jammed. Also check the pressure gauge on the filter to see if water is being pumped or not. But don't overlook the possibility that gauges can sometime stick in the zero flow position. Give the gauge a light tap to dislodge the needle. If this is not the case, put your hand over an inlet port in the pool and check the water flow. Confusion can sometimes arise with one of the clear, see-through lids on a pump strainer because it is often hard to detect water movement when the pump is on. If the water is clear and neither air nor debris are entering the strainer, the clear water will not show obvious signs of movement. Double-check by feeling the flow from the outlet into the pool.

If the pump is running but not pumping water, and you've checked and cleaned the pump strainer and skimmer box and the inlet and outlet lines are open, check and tighten any loose bolts and fittings on the suction side of the pump. Make sure the strainer is filled with water. Be sure to bleed the air from the filter casing after starting the pump. In the event that these checks and the checks for cavitation (below) do not reveal a simple solution, consult a

> If the motor is allowed to run with noisy bearings, they will eventually seize, melting the collar, and the only answer will be a new motor.

pool serviceman before you go any further.

Cavitation. The majority of pump problems are caused by air leaks (cavitation) in the suction line. Cavitation, put simply, is when the pump is trying to circulate more water than is available in the pipe. This can cause water to turn to vapor, forming vapor pockets near the impeller. This results in excessive pump noise because the pump strains to bring in more water than is available to it, caused either by a partially blocked inlet pipe or one that is too small in diameter for the pump. If the water line is not obstructed, a pool technician would more than likely attach a vacuum gauge to the leaf strainer to test for cavitation. The solution (without replacing the inlet line) is to cut down the flow rate, thereby reducing the amount of vacuum created by the pump.

Sounds play an important part in pump malfunction diagnosis. If there is an air leak on the inlet side of the pump, either through a loose strainer lid, worn gasket, or worn O-rings, the pumping rate will tend to be uneven. The pump may run well for a time, then change sound and speed as air is drawn in. Then, as the air is expelled, the pump starts working again. Often, in this case, the strainer or pot will be only half-filled with water—the pump will gurgle, strain, and air will be pumped into the filter tank. Look for a poorly seated strainer pot lid, check for loose or damaged fittings, or a crack or split in the pipes or flexible inlet line. If these check out okay, chances are the problem lies with worn O-rings or a damaged water seal.

If, on the other hand, the problem is cavitation caused by an obstruction in the suction line, the pump tends to labor on a more constant note than it does when air is leaking in. This is your clue to check for an obstruction on the inlet side—at the skimmer box, in the strainer pot, through a partially closed inlet valve

or partially blocked pipe, or an air lock in the pump or inlet line. If neither you nor a repair company can find the obstruction or source of the problem, the final resort will be to buy a new pump.

It is also possible for pool pumps to be mounted so that the discharge opening or outlet to the filter is pointing toward the bottom of the pump. If this is the case, the pump should be remounted with the outlet pointing toward the top of the pump, because air can become trapped in the top half of the pump body and cause continual problems, leading to eventual pump failure.

One other check you can make for cavitation is to restrict the outlet flow from the pump, either by slowly closing the gate valve (if fitted) or slowing down the flow from the pool inlet with a piece of wood or plastic or your hand. As pressure increases, the cavitation noise will disappear. Air leaks can occur if the suction and return lines to the pool are too short or if the piping is too large for the pump capacity. One way to handle this, without the expensive job of replacing the pipes, is to put a gate valve on the outlet line between the filter and the pool. The gate valve can then be partially closed until cavitation ceases. If allowed to continue, cavitation can damage both the impeller and bearings.

The Five Most Common Pump Problems

1. **Cavitation** caused by a restriction in the suction line, such as a blocked leaf strainer on the pump, or a blocked skimmer inlet.

2. An **air leak** in the suction line can be trouble. This can result from faulty or worn seals and pipe joints, or a pool level that is so low it allows air to be sucked in through the skimmer. Air in the suction line becomes trapped inside the pump, reducing efficiency.

3. A **worn mechanical seal** between the pump and motor that al-

Cavitation, put simply, is when the pump is trying to circulate more water than is available in the pipe.

Sounds play an important part in pump malfunction diagnosis.

WHAT COLOR IS YOUR SWIMMING POOL?

lows air to be sucked into the pump, decreasing pump efficiency.

4. The **impeller is worn.** The edges of the impeller vanes can be worn down, particularly if you live in a dusty or sandy area and large quantities of fine gritty dust are vacuumed from the floor of the pool. Sometimes this grit can lodge between the vanes and back plate, damaging both. This wear can reduce the efficiency of the pump. The solution is to replace the impeller and, if necessary, the wear plate.

5. **Fouling of the impeller** with hair, lint, or leaves. Sometimes you can remove the obstruction by taking the lid off the leaf strainer and reaching through to the impeller with your fingers. *But first be sure to turn off the power to the pump.*

In the event of breakdown or mechanical failure, pump and motor repair can be complicated. This chapter has covered only the most elementary of pump repairs. Should you want to know more about this mechanical component, read the maintenance manual that came with it, or ask at a pool service store about other maintenance books or pamphlets on this subject.

6 • Pool Heaters

A swimming pool heater can extend the swimming season from early spring until late fall. In many areas of the country a pool heater can provide year-round swimming. There are four heating systems — gas-fired, oil, electric, and solar. Your choice will depend on which part of the country you live in and the kind of use your pool gets. In some parts of the nation, natural gas is cheaper than electricity and vice versa. If you are considering building a pool, it is cheaper to install the heater while building than to add it later on. Even if you don't think you want a heater now, it would be smart to have the builder install heater inlet and outlet lines, in case you change your mind later.

HEATER OPTIONS

It used to be that gas or oil-fired heaters were more efficient than electrical units. But manufacturers have developed some remarkably efficient electrical units, and cost/efficiency comparison data is readily available from manufacturers and dealers. Solar heaters can deliver nearly cost-free operation, but the initial investment can be considerable and it is absolutely critical that they be correctly installed by a solar-heating contractor who knows the business.

When it comes to pool heaters, bigger is better — to a point. The pool consumes the same amount of heat regardless of whether it is supplied quickly or over an extended period of time. If the heater is too small, the water loses too much heat during the warming-up period and the small heater can end up using more energy than a larger unit and never get the pool up to the temperature you want. The only restriction to buying an oversize heater is the initial cost of the unit itself.

What you want is a heater large enough to get the water temperature up to a comfortable level — 75°F to 78°F (24°C to 26°C) — quickly. The heater will then close down and won't come back on until the temperature has dropped below the established level. Medical authorities recommend water temperature of 78°F for recreational swimming. Remember, for every additional degree of pool water temperature, the energy requirement jumps significantly — in some cases, as much as 10 percent for each degree above 78°F.

Medical authorities recommend water temperature of 78°F for recreational swimming. Remember, for every additional degree of water temperature, the energy requirement jumps significantly — in some cases, as much as 10 percent for each degree above 78°F.

The choice of heater styles and types, and the sophistication of controls, make selection difficult. Modern pool heaters offer convertibility from electric to either natural gas or propane (LP) gas, pull-out circuit board controls, and venting for either enclosed or outdoor installation. Some have pilot lights and others offer electronic ignition that eliminates the need for a pilot light. Some heaters feature such innovations as automatic shut-off pressure switches and electronic controls that can be operated from inside the house by remote control. What follows is a discussion of things a pool owner should know before a pool heater is chosen and installed.

A dealer, distributor, or pool builder should already have comparative operation figures and energy costs for natural gas, LP gas, oil, and electric heaters. Heater manufacturers supply detailed heater-sizing charts and installation instructions. The choice will depend on four things: first, your preference for fuel; sec-

ond, operating costs in your area; third, state and local regulations regarding pool heaters; and fourth, the physical conditions existing at your pool.

Do your research first: determine what the heating needs are for your pool, how much you want to spend to have a heater installed, how much you want to spend annually to operate it, and what kind of system your pool area can accommodate. With these observations in hand, have a pool dealer come by, inspect your pool, and get his advice. He will look to see if there is enough room around the pump and filter area to fit the required pipes and valves, and if there is enough room for the heater itself. He will also check to see where the return lines from the filter to the pool are located. For efficient heating, return inlets should be positioned low down on the wall or else angled to direct hot water to the lowest part of the pool. Otherwise, the surface water may be heated (because heat rises) but the

Illustration by Chrysalis Design Group

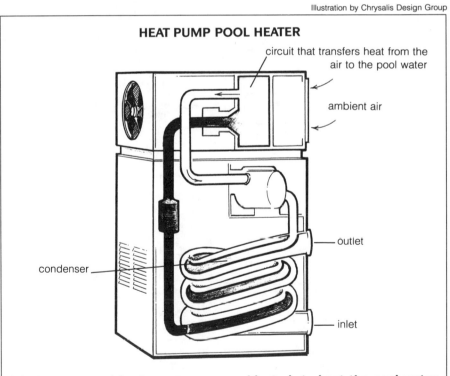

HEAT PUMP POOL HEATER

circuit that transfers heat from the air to the pool water

ambient air

condenser

outlet

inlet

A heat pump pool heater uses warm ambient air to heat the pool water being filtered through it, and therefore is not recommended for colder climates.

deeper water will remain cold. And, because heat loss occurs at the water surface of the pool, it is inefficient to keep pumping heated water into the surface layers. Ask the builder or dealer to check this for you, and whether he would advise that the inlet be repositioned if heat is not being evenly distributed.

The pool dealer or builder will also check to see if the interconnecting pipes from the heater to the pool are exposed to cold winds. If so, the pipes and fittings should be insulated. The pump and filter must also be in good condition. Air leaks on the suction side of the pump can let air into the heater—a major source of problems in pool heaters. The pump and filter must be in good enough condition and powerful enough to handle the extra head pressure the heater adds to the system—this is particularly critical when a solar installation is being considered.

Heat Loss

Heat loss should be a consideration of the dealer or builder installing the heater. Heat-loss prevention should definitely be of concern to you, as a pool owner, because you can reduce the costs of heating a pool by as much as 50 to 70 percent, depending on the area you live in. Wind is a major factor in heat loss. If your pool is subject to cool breezes, a large amount of heat will be lost. This can be reduced considerably by sheltering the pool with a louvered or basketweave fence, thick hedge, or other windbreak, but

Illustration by Chrysalis Design Group

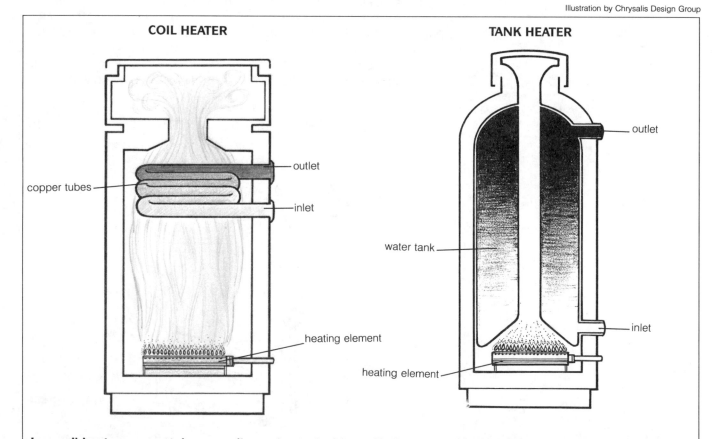

COIL HEATER

copper tubes

outlet

inlet

heating element

In a coil heater copper tubes or coils are heated with electricity or an open flame, and that warmth is transferred to the pool water being pumped through the system.

TANK HEATER

outlet

water tank

inlet

heating element

Similar to a residential hot-water heater, pool tank heaters use an open flame to heat a large tank of water. Tank heaters take a long time to warm up and a long time to replenish the warm water supply, and are only recommended for small pools.

WHAT COLOR IS YOUR SWIMMING POOL?

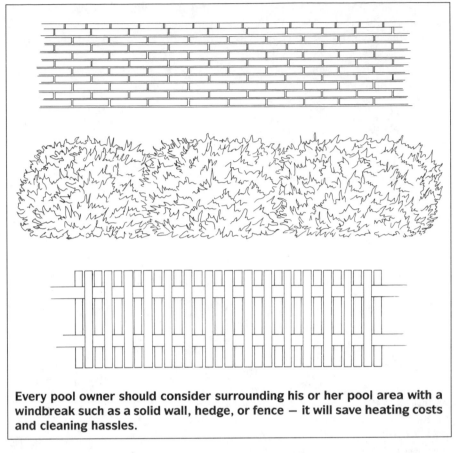

Every pool owner should consider surrounding his or her pool area with a windbreak such as a solid wall, hedge, or fence — it will save heating costs and cleaning hassles.

There are many other ways to reduce the overall energy costs of operating your pool such as proper sizing and selection of a pump and filter, and designing an efficient circulation system.

the most common solution is to install a pool cover. An efficient heater, pool cover, and windbreak could save you a significant amount in energy costs.

A wall, fence, cabana or other structure acting as a wind barrier can reduce heating costs significantly. A drop in wind velocity of only a few miles per hour, even in a light breeze, can significantly reduce heat loss while the pool is uncovered. The difference between no wind across the surface of the pool and a breeze of 7 miles per hour can mean a 400 percent increase in heating cost. If vacationing for 2 weeks or longer, turn the heater off completely, including the pilot light, if so equipped.

There are many other ways to reduce the overall energy costs of operating your pool such as proper sizing and selection of a pump and filter, and designing an efficient circulation system. You can also cut down on filtering time by regular vacuuming and making sure the filter does not continue to operate after the water is clean.

When using a heater, realize that the water may feel chilly at first if you keep it at the recommended 78°F (26°C). The temptation is to set the heater thermostat higher, but swimmers will find the water quite comfortable in a short time and will probably have finished their swim before the pool heater can raise the water temperature even one-half a degree. Once you've set the thermostat, forbid tampering with it. You might consider a setscrew to lock it in place.

According to studies by the NSPI, predetermination of your swimming season can save at least 33 percent of all energy typically used to operate the pool. Be realistic about this. Do you really use your pool every day during the Northeastern swimming season; or every day in November or December, or in March or April in the Southwest and West? If swimming dwindles to weekends and other special occasions during certain months, it will require less energy to heat your swimming pool for the weekend than to keep it heated all week. You can use the thermostat as a switch or install an ON/OFF switch on the heater. Bear in mind that the typical pool heater takes about 1 hour to raise pool temperature 1 degree, so allow enough time for the water to reach a comfortable swimming temperature.

All told, there is a wide range of measures you can take to reduce heat loss from the pool and thereby cut energy costs. In addition to windbreaks and covers, circulation pipes and equipment can be insulated. It is also possible, in colder climates, to have the pool shell itself insulated against the cold from the surrounding earth, although you would have to compare the additional cost against possible heat savings. At this time, I am not aware of any objective research into such savings, but your local pool builder may have some information for you.

Enclosing the pump, filter, and heater in a suitable shed will also cut down on heat loss, as well as protect the equipment from the weather and windblown dust and leaves. But remember, good ventilation is essential for safe and efficient heater operation. Observe manufacturer's warnings about clearance and ventilation.

Heater Operation in a New Pool

For a newly-constructed pool, don't operate the heater until the pool surfaces and water have been thoroughly cleaned and the water correctly balanced. Construction sediment in a new pool will rapidly fill the filter, which necessitates frequent backwashing, and the resulting pressure variations in the system could cause the heater to cycle on

and off rapidly. This won't damage the heater, but it is inefficient and uneconomical. It is far better to let the filter system thoroughly cleanse the pool before turning on the heating system.

SOLAR HEATING

There are an estimated 100,000 to 150,000 solar-heated swimming pools in the United States today. The biggest drawback to widespread use of solar heating for swimming pools is the initial cost. Although solar may offer "free energy" from the sun, it is going to cost you a great deal to install a basic solar heating system. Depending on how much use you get from your pool, the payback in energy savings could take up to 10 years. But the biggest advantage is that the purchase of a solar heating system effectively freezes most of your future pool heating expenses. What that expense would have been then becomes the payment of interest on any debt incurred to buy the system. And, of course, solar heating is non-polluting and environmentally acceptable.

This discussion of solar pool heating is primarily concerned with *active solar heating* systems; such a system uses collectors to capture the sun's heat, and through it the pool water is pumped, heated, and returned to the pool. *Passive solar heating* systems include pool enclosures and translucent and bubble plastic pool covers that "collect" heat from the sun and transfer that heat to the water. A slight increase in solar heating effect can be obtained by painting the floor and walls of the pool in dark colors which will better absorb heat from the sun.

Choosing a solar heating system. Because solar radiation varies at each installation site, as does the space available to mount the panels and the amount of heat required,

Bear in mind that the typical pool heater takes about 1 hour to raise pool temperature 1 degree, so allow enough time for the water to reach a comfortable swimming temperature.

Enclosing the pump, filter, and heater in a suitable shed will also cut down on heat loss, as well as protect the equipment from the weather and windblown dust and leaves.

> The difference in cost between an unglazed and glazed collector panel system is considerable. Unglazed plastic or copper collectors cost between $5 and $20 per square foot less than glazed copper collectors. The difference lies in the fact that glazed collectors are more efficient convertors of the sun's energy.

only broad recommendations are provided here.

If you are considering solar heating check with several companies who have installed solar heating systems on other pools in your area. These would include pool builders, solar heating companies, and pool service companies. Some companies utilize computer programs to calculate the heat load data needed to correctly design a solar system for each particular pool and location. Such programs also provide reasonably accurate predictions of energy savings compared to conventional heating systems. Reputable companies will provide the names of pool owners for whom they have installed a solar system. Most solar owners are happy to talk about their systems. If they will let you see the installation, so much the better. You don't want to wait until the system is installed to find out that the collectors mar the appearance of your house or backyard.

The difference in cost between an *unglazed* and *glazed* collector panel system is considerable. Unglazed plastic or copper collectors cost between $5 and $20 per square foot less than glazed copper collectors. The difference lies in the fact that glazed collectors are more efficient convertors of the sun's energy. An unglazed solar panel system, for instance, when correctly installed, will collect about 50,000 to 150,000 BTUs per square foot of collector surface per swimming season. (BTU stands for British Thermal Unit, which is the amount of heat required to raise the temperature of 1 pound of water 1°F per hour.) A glazed collector system, on the other hand, will collect about 150,000 to 450,000 BTUs per square foot of collector per swimming season.

Which system you select depends on a number of factors: where you live, how close to true south the panels can be located, the temperature of the water you prefer, and how many months of comfortable swim-ming you want. Unglazed collectors work well in the warmer, sheltered areas of the Southwest, but if you live in the Midwest or East, glazed collectors will have to be used if you want the water to be warmer than the ambient air temperature—this will, of course, extend the swimming season. The collector area needed will probably equal 50 to 75 percent of the square footage of your pool, whatever system you use. The minimum figure is 50 percent and the maximum figure depends on where you live. In the colder areas of the nation, the panels would probably have to equal the area of the pool, or even 1½ times the surface area of the pool in order to heat the water during cold months.

Active Solar Heating

The operation of active solar heating is quite simple. A series of solar collector panels are mounted on a roof or at ground level, facing as close to true south as possible and angled toward the sun. The panels are connected by pipes to the outlet side of the pool filter pump. Pool water is pumped to the collectors, where it is heated by the sun's radiation as it travels through a series of small-diameter plastic or copper tubes, then returned to the pool.

Unglazed plastic panels. Low-cost solar pool heating systems use relatively inexpensive panels made of black rubber, composition rubber, or plastic tubing or channels, without insulation or glazing. Because these collectors are designed for situations where the pool temperature has to be raised only a few degrees, plastic (or PVC) pipes and fittings can be used for the supply and return lines. So, the entire installation is far less expensive than the glazed panels and copper pipes necessary for domestic solar water heating systems, or ones used for spas or hot tubs. The drawback, though, is that you will need a lot more of the unglazed plastic collectors than with a

Illustration by Chrysalis Design Group

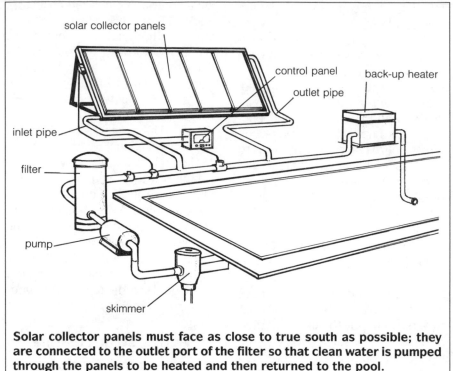

solar collector panels

control panel

back-up heater

outlet pipe

inlet pipe

filter

pump

skimmer

Solar collector panels must face as close to true south as possible; they are connected to the outlet port of the filter so that clean water is pumped through the panels to be heated and then returned to the pool.

glazed collector system. In a 29,000 gallon pool, for instance, you would need space to mount about 16 unglazed plastic panels, which would cover most of your roof space. Alternatively, you can mount them on frames, or on a south-facing slope of earth. They must face true south at the correct angle for your latitude; and they must be higher than the pool so they can be drained when freezing temperatures occur. The panels also must be supported in the back by a flat surface of some kind and held in place in such a way that they will not rub against anything during the expansion and contraction that takes place. If not, the expansion and contraction can damage the panels.

Glazed panels. Why would anyone opt for the much more expensive glazed system? There may not be an option. The low-temperature unglazed collector system is best suited to situations in which the pool water does not need to be heated more than 5° Fahrenheit above the average ambient air temperature

range. As the air temperature drops below the 5-degree range—for example, air temperature is 72°F (22°C) and pool temperature is 77°F (25°C)—the performance of the unglazed collector drops off sharply. When you want to heat the pool water over a wider range, say a 10-degree spread between pool water temperature and air temperature— air temperature is 65°F (18°C) and water temperature is 75°F (24°C)— it will take a glazed system to do so.

Because glazed panels generate hot water faster, and with less panel space, they are the only choice if you wish to heat a pool in conjunction with a spa or hot tub, or with your domestic hot water supply. Because of the much higher temperatures generated, some manufacturers strongly recommend copper pipes be used. One word of caution: with some glazed solar panels, there have been problems with high temperatures breaking down the sanitizing chemicals in the pool water. Needless to say, with copper collectors and pipes, balanced water is absolutely essential. Unbalanced

The low-temperature unglazed collector system is best suited to situations in which the pool water does not need to be heated more than 5°F above the average ambient air temperature range.

> Most heaters have an automatic overload switch that shuts off the heater when the water supply falls below an adequate level.

> Good ventilation is also essential to safe and efficient operation of a heater. Stackless (no chimney) heaters should be installed at least 8 feet away from doors or windows to prevent carbon monoxide from the heater being sucked into the house.

water can quickly corrode or deposit scale in the collectors, severely reducing efficiency and in extreme cases ruining the system. This is another point in favor of the plastic-panel systems.

A solar pool heating system should also have thermostatically controlled diverter valves to close the pipes to the pool whenever the temperature of the heated water from collectors is lower than the pool water temperature. Otherwise, you'll be cooling the water in the pool, not heating it. This also requires that there be heat sensing units in the pool and at the collector panels, and a differential thermostat control to operate the diverter valves.

Frankly, if you're going to invest in a solar system, get the best quality system you can afford and, most important of all, have it designed and installed by true experts in solar pool heating systems. Get recommendations from NSPI or pool owners in your area who have solar heating. Solar is still a young and growing industry, and there are a number of untrained and unlicensed operators at work. Just because a solar heating company installs domestic hot water systems does not mean they know anything about pool systems. These are completely different areas of expertise.

HEATER MAINTENANCE

Fortunately, most pool heaters require little maintenance if correctly installed and if the connected equipment (pump and filter) are correctly maintained. Manufacturers recommend at least an annual inspection by a competent pool technician. Shortly before opening the pool is a good time to check the heater's condition if you had shut down the pool for the winter. When using a heater, correct water treatment is essential. The water should be kept in a balanced condition as much as possi-

ble to protect the heater mechanism. Unbalanced water can seriously reduce heater efficiency in a relatively short period of time, and severely imbalanced water can effectively destroy a heater in the course of one season through scale buildup and calcification.

Good ventilation is also essential to safe and efficient operation of a heater. Stackless (no chimney) heaters should be installed at least 8 feet away from doors or windows to prevent carbon monoxide from the heater being sucked into the house. Also, a heater that is placed too close to a high wall can be subject to swirling, downdraft winds that will extinguish the pilot. The heater should be at least 3 feet away from such a wall. Don't allow leaves and other debris to accumulate near the heater. Debris and dust can block the vents, reducing efficiency. The vents and the area around the bottom of the heater should be cleaned regularly.

Troubleshooting Pool Heaters

If the heater is not working correctly or isn't working at all, check the obvious first. Has the fuel supply been turned off or, if it is an electric heater, has the breaker tripped or the fuse blown? If the fuel supply seems sufficient, there may not be enough water reaching the heater. Most heaters have an automatic overload switch that shuts off the heater when the water supply falls below an adequate level. In addition, check for leaves and debris blocking the skimmer, the leaf strainer on the pump, a dirty filter, or a valve that someone may have turned off.

The most common problem is that the pilot light has gone out. New electronic ignition heaters don't have a pilot light. An ignition source is activated each time the heater is turned or cycles on. Check for sparking at the pilot burner electrode. If not, check the attached fuse. The most common reason for the pilot light not coming on is air in the line. On a gas heater, test for this by turning on the gas supply until the air is purged from the line and you can smell gas at the pilot. You should never light a pilot with your head close to the heater. And stand well back until the burners light.

If the heater still doesn't fire up, the problem is most likely the injector system of an oil-fired heater, the gas regulator in a gas heater, or an electrical fault in an electric heater. Don't think twice about it—call in a qualified repairman to solve the problem. To do otherwise will not only void your warranty, but may void any insurance you carry.

One test you can make is to look at the color of the pilot light on a gas heater. If the flame is "lazy" and yellow in color, there could be a problem with the gas pressure, or the pilot hole may be clogged with soot or insects. Don't clean the pilot with a wire brush—it could produce a spark and ignite soot in the heater, which is flammable. Pilot valves should be cleaned with compressed air or a soft bristle brush. If the pilot light keeps cycling on and off, it is probably a faulty pressure switch. Again, call in a factory-trained representative. Inexpert tinkering can be dangerous and, at the least, more expensive in the long run than calling in a qualified expert.

The most common reason for the pilot light not coming on is in the air in the line.

7 • Pool Covers

If you have just bought or installed a pool, probably the last thing on your mind is covering it up. When you realize just how much debris and dust a rain storm or high wind can deposit into your pool—and how much work it takes to get that stuff out—you will understand why pool covers are one of the most frequently recommended pool accessories. Pool covers range from relatively inexpensive (thin gauge) vinyl, polyethelene, and laminated polyesters to more expensive, heavy gauge vinyl, polyethylene, vinyl laminates, and polypropylene mesh. Covers do more than keep out leaves and debris. They also reduce water loss through evaporation, reduce chemical loss, help to retain heat, and with solar or thermal pool covers actually raise the water temperature through a passive solar heat collection.

Generally speaking, covers are grouped under solar or thermal covers (blankets), winter covers, automatic (rigid) covers, and safety covers. According to the manufacturers, a safety cover is one that, when installed, can be walked on by children, pets, and adults without the danger of falling through into the water. Safety covers are also fitted and/or tied down so that pets and

small children cannot wiggle under the cover and get into the water. The majority of winter covers and solar/thermal covers are not fastened in this way, nor are they designed to support someone foolish enough to try and walk on them. At the top end of the line are automatic rigid covers, which are usually made of aluminum and fiberglass panels that seal off the pool completely. When the pool is in use they can be folded back to make windbreaks or raised over the pool like a patio roof. The fiberglass construction also allows passive solar heating of the water.

When you are in the market for a pool cover the best course of action is to visit local pool builders and pool supply store showrooms and review the manufacturer's literature. Determine the ease of handling and durability of pool covers that are suitable to your area. Ask for recommendations as to quality and the strength of warranties offered by manufacturers and distributors (usually 3 to 5 years).

Solar Covers

Solar (or thermal) covers are usually made of vinyl or polyethylene and contain trapped air bubbles that

FIGURE 7.1

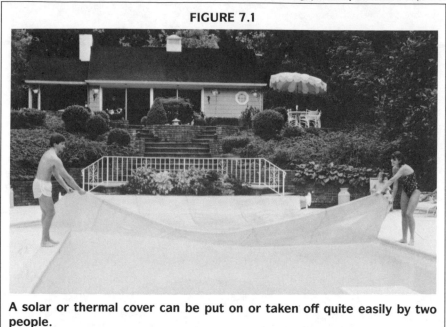

A solar or thermal cover can be put on or taken off quite easily by two people.

enable such a cover to float on the pool surface and increase the passive solar heating effect by trapping the sun's radiation beneath it (Figure 7.1). They can be put on and taken off quite readily by two people, or you can step up to a hand-cranked pool cover on a reel or one driven by an electric motor. Manufacturers claim that such covers can pay for themselves through energy and pool chemical savings. Some claim their covers reduce pool heating costs by up to 70 percent, others claim that heat gain during daylight hours is increased by 25 to 35 percent or more, and that the savings in chemicals and reduced pool cleaning are substantial. You will have to judge the validity of these claims yourself. Nevertheless, solar covers do prevent heat loss overnight and on cooler days, they do heat the water on sunny days, and they do cut down on water and chemical loss.

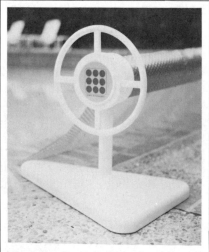

Most pool covers come on a reel that is either hand cranked or motor driven.

Solar covers *do* prevent heat loss overnight and on cooler days, they *do* heat the water on sunny days, and they *do* cut down on water and chemical loss.

Winter Covers

As the name suggests, winter covers are designed to protect the pool over the winter months when it is not in use. Obviously, they are far more popular (and necessary) in colder regions of the country than in the South or Southwest where pools are often used year-round. Winter covers are usually made of heavy gauge vinyl or vinyl laminations, specially reinforced and treated to resist scuffing and wear from ice, sun, and snow (Figure 7.2). The most common method of tying down winter covers is with built-in or separate water bags or water tube anchors, about 8 or 10 feet

No matter what kind of pool cover or blanket you choose *never* use the pool with a blanket or cover partially or completely in place.

long. Filled with water or sand they secure the covers around the edge of the pool.

Safety Covers

Usually made of close-woven, strong polypropylene mesh with strong cover straps, safety covers are tied securely around the pool with flush-mounted anchors (Figure 7.3). A floating vinyl or polyethylene solar cover is recommended for use beneath the safety cover to keep out fine debris and dust which can filter through the woven mesh. Such covers need to be initially installed by the manufacturer or distributor and are often guaranteed for up to 10 or 15 years. Even though one manufacturer claims his safety covers have a snow-load capacity of 60,000 pounds, it would be wise to occasionally clear away snow to relieve the strain on the cover straps and fittings. Some safety covers offer fastening or tie-down systems with a lock mechanism that cannot be bypassed by unauthorized visitors. If safety is your prime consideration, such covers are worth investigating.

To keep things simple, I've also included automatic rigid covers under safety covers. Two main types are available. One runs on a concealed track system on the underside of the deck coping and when not in use rolls up on an automatic roller system. The cover is made of rigid slats of vinyl. Such covers must be custom-made and installed. The other type consists of rigid fiberglass panels on an aluminum frame. These can be hinged and folded back to form windbreaks, or totally removed. Another style of rigid-type cover is a one-piece cover, which is raised or lowered on slim columns around the pool perimeter. When raised for swimming, the cover acts as a kind of solar patio roof. When lowered, both types have all the virtues of solar covers in their ability to conserve heat, cut down on water and chemical loss, and act as passive solar heaters.

No matter what kind of pool cover or blanket you choose *never* use the pool with a blanket or cover partially

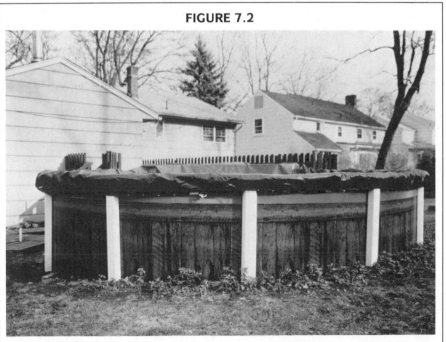

FIGURE 7.2

This above-ground winter cover is made of heavy vinyl and has been securely tied in place to prevent snow, ice, and debris from fouling the pool surface.

FIGURE 7.3

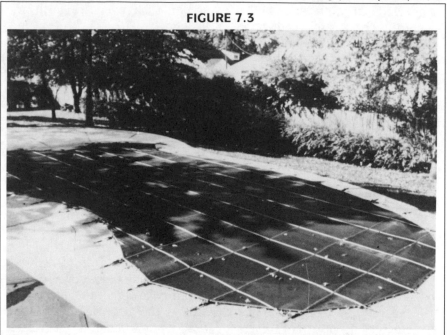

Safety covers are often custom fitted and feature tiedowns that are fastened flush with the pool deck. More than just protection from leaves and dirt, a safety cover is intended to support the weight of any person who might mistakenly step onto it.

or completely in place. To do so is to invite disaster, because swimmers could become disoriented or panic if they find themselves under the cover.

Pool covers are relatively inexpensive, can be made to fit almost any pool shape, and most can be applied or removed by one person. Properly cared for, they will last for years and pay for themselves in freedom from maintenance hassles and savings on your first year's utility bills.

8 • Pool Cleaning

Because it is much easier to remove debris while it is on the surface, many pool owners make it a habit to skim the pool surface every day.

To keep your pool clean and inviting, and to reduce the load on the filter, a regular cleaning schedule is essential. There is no established pattern for pool cleaning, but the one used by many pool service companies is a good model.

1. Test the water for residual chlorine level, pH, total alkalinity, and calcium hardness, but don't add chemicals to the water until cleaning and vacuuming have been completed.

2. Skim all leaves and debris from the water surface with a leaf skimmer. A leaf skimmer is an aluminum, stainless-steel, or plastic frame with a mesh skimming net. Skimmers are designed to attach to a single-piece or telescopic aluminum handle that also fits the vacuum cleaner and cleaning brushes. Handles range in length from 8 to 16 feet. A leaf skimmer can also be used to pick up debris from the pool bottom. Because it is much easier to remove debris while it is on the surface, many pool owners make it a habit to skim the pool surface every day.

3. Clean the tile and walls. A sponge or rag with regular household scouring powder will remove the scum at the waterline, though you can buy special tile cleaners for use with a brush. Light scale can be removed with a soft pumice stone block, if you take care not to scratch the tile surface. Sometimes a razor blade is effective. But don't use steel wool—steel particles can become embedded in the grout and will stain it. Persistent scale is a sign that water is seriously out of balance. Correct it as described on pages 16-18, or call in professional help. Don't let this imbalance persist or it will damage not only the pool surfaces, but the equipment as well.

4. Brush the pool walls. A nylon brush is tough enough to remove dirt on fiberglass or vinyl-liner pools. On a plastered concrete pool, use a stainless steel brush to remove stubborn dirt and algae growth. Brush the walls from the top down to the floor of the pool so that the vacuum cleaner can collect it. Start brushing at the shallow end and work towards the deep end. Brushing dirt toward the main drain will allow some of it to be pulled into the filter system during this process.

5. Clean out the strainer basket in the skimmer box and the pump's leaf strainer regularly.

6. Vacuum the pool. There are two basic types of nonautomatic pool vacuum cleaners. One type works

from the vacuum inlet in the skimmer or a vacuum fitting in the pool wall. The other type is called a jet cleaner. It uses the pressure from a garden hose connected to the cleaner head. A full discussion of vacuum equipment and procedures appears on the following pages.

7. Backwash the filter when it is indicated and only operate it when it is in good working condition.

8. Add the necessary chemicals to maintain the water in a safe and balanced condition. See chapter 3 for a more complete discussion of water treatment.

9. Brush or hose down the coping and deck. Always sweep or spray away from the pool to prevent dust and silt from being washed or brushed into the pool water. A weak (5 percent) solution of chlorine and water to occasionally wash down decking during summer months will kill bacteria and prevent the spread of infections such as athlete's foot.

BASIC EQUIPMENT AND PROCEDURES

Basic pool-cleaning equipment includes a pool vacuum cleaner, a leaf skimmer, and one or two brush heads. These are the essential pieces of equipment, but you can add timesaving items if you wish. Manufacturers are constantly developing new timesaving pieces of equipment; your local pool supply dealers should have catalogs available.

Vacuum Cleaners

The most common type of non-automatic vacuum cleaner consists of a cleaning head on wheels—it comes equipped with or without a brush; or the head may be equipped only with a brush. The wheeled type without brushes is designed for vinyl-liner or fiberglass pools. All brush-type vacuum heads will do a more thorough job of cleaning tacky debris on the pool bottom.

If you have a pool with a rough plaster finish, the wheel-and-brush-head vacuum cleaner is what you need. The wheeled head without brushes will not always remove dirt lodged in a rough plaster surface. You could use an all-brush head on a plaster pool, but make sure the brushes are replaceable because they will wear down rapidly. Also, look for a vacuum head with some weight to it. A lightweight head will tend to float off the pool bottom near the end of an outward sweep.

The wheel-and-brush-type of vacuum connects directly to the pool's filter system, either through a vacuum fitting located in the skimmer box or in the pool wall. The filter system draws water and debris through the vacuum head and into the filter, returning clean water to the pool. The vacuum head is connected to the vacuum fitting by a long hose, and the head is pushed along the bottom of the pool by means of a long pole—usually the same pole used for the leaf skimmer and pool brushes.

The other type of nonautomatic pool vacuum is called a jet cleaner. It doesn't use the pool filter system—a garden hose is used to create the vacuum action at the cleaner head. The hose can be attached to a garden faucet, but it should be at least ¾ of an inch in diameter and provide good pressure (about 40 pounds pressure minimum at the faucet). Water is forced into the throat of the suction head. This creates water flow from the vacuum head up into a cotton or synthetic-weave bag. Leaves, dust, and debris are caught in the filter bag, allowing clean water to pass through. When vacuuming is completed, the filter bag is removed and emptied. One advantage of a jet cleaner is that it removes leaves better than a standard vacuum cleaner and filter combination, but it is not as efficient at picking up fine dirt particles. Another advantage is that the jet cleaner does not run heavy loads

The most common type of nonautomatic vacuum cleaner consists of a cleaning head on wheels—it comes equipped with or without a brush.

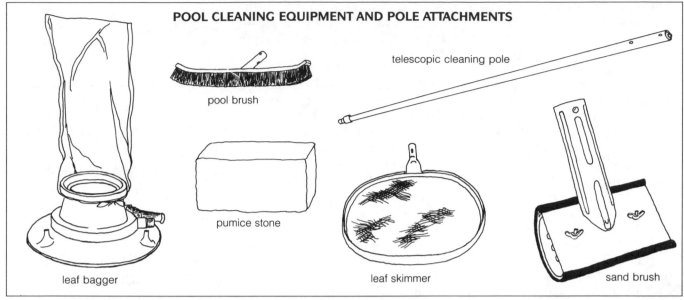

POOL CLEANING EQUIPMENT AND POLE ATTACHMENTS

telescopic cleaning pole

pool brush

pumice stone

leaf bagger

leaf skimmer

sand brush

of dirt and debris through the filter system.

When using pool vacuum cleaners, you might find it useful to follow the procedure outlined below.

The night before you plan to vacuum, turn off the filter system. This will allow suspended dirt or dust particles to fall to the bottom of the pool.

If the filter system needs backwashing, do this before vacuuming or it will quickly load up and considerably reduce the efficiency of the vacuum cleaner.

Check that the water level in the pool is above the vacuum inlet fitting or skimmer inlet fitting, depending on which is used. You must avoid getting air into the inlet line, and thus into the water pump and filter. Air in the vacuum line is the most common reason that a vacuum won't work.

Follow the procedure outlined in the vacuum manufacturer's owner's manual regarding operation. The usual procedure, if you're using a special vacuum fitting line, is to close the main suction valve and skimmer valves to provide maximum suction on the vacuum cleaner line. If using a vacuum line in the skimmer box, close off the main drain suction line.

Attach the vacuum handle and one end of the vacuum hose to the vacuum head. Place the vacuum head in the pool and let it drop to the bottom. Take the other end of the vacuum hose and hold it against the return line from the filter to the pool. The water pressure flowing into the hose will drive out the air. Alternatively, you can put the vacuum head in the pool and slowly feed the hose into the water until it is completely filled with water. It is important not to have any air in the hose or to let the vacuum head rise above the water surface. Air in the hose, or sucked in through the head, can cause the pump to lose its prime.

If using the skimmer box, attach the vacuum plate provided with the skimmer box. The plate is usually made of molded plastic with some type of gasket to act as a seal. It is used to cover the main drain connection and to increase vacuum suction. Be sure the plate sits flat; if it doesn't, the suction will try to flatten the plate and could crack it. Connect the vacuum hose to the plate quickly. Once the vacuum plate is in place, the increased suction will start to form a vortex, which can draw air into the suction line. The suction line in the skimmer box is

The usual procedure, if you're using a special vacuum fitting line, is to close the main suction valve and skimmer valves to provide maximum suction on the vacuum cleaner line.

usually easy to recognize because it lies below the level of the basket. If using a special vacuum fitting in the pool, connect the end of the hose to the fitting.

Begin vacuuming, starting at the shallow end and working toward the deep end. You will find it more efficient to vacuum around the edges first, moving the vacuum head parallel to the walls of the pool, with the head close against the wall. When the edges are clean, then start vacuuming across the pool. Use slow, even strokes. If you push the head too fast it will disperse the dirt into the water instead of sucking it up.

When finished vacuuming, clean out the skimmer basket and pump's leaf strainer, and backwash the filter if indicated. Then return the valves to their normal operating positions.

If vacuum efficiency starts to drop, check and clean the skimmer basket. If this doesn't improve performance, check the pump's leaf strainer and clean it out. Also check the pressure at the filter, and backwash if needed. Most filters have an air bleed valve on the tank. Periodically bleed any accumulated air as you vacuum if you find it necessary.

If there is an extremely heavy dirt load in the pool, as may happen after a heavy rain or dusty winds, it will quickly overload the filter. To avoid this situation you can switch the filter to waste, or put it in the backwash mode until the majority of the dirt has been vacuumed.

Don't spend too much time at this because you're draining water from the pool, which will have to be replaced.

If dirt accumulation in the pool is light, an alternative to vacuuming is to brush the walls of the pool the day before you intend to vacuum. The brushed dirt will settle on the pool bottom, and you may be able to simply brush the dirt into the main drain while the filter system is on. When doing this, both the skimmer and vacuum lines should be closed so that the main drain in the bottom of the pool is operating at maximum suction. Again, brush from the shallow end toward the deep end, where the main drain is located. Use slow, even strokes to minimize the chances of dirt being swirled up from the pool bottom and suspended in the water.

Automatic Pool Cleaners

Automatic pool cleaning systems can be built into a pool during construction, but the most popular are portable automatic pool cleaners or pool sweeps, which can be purchased after the pool is built. There are numerous manufacturers of portable automatic pool cleaners, all of which are effective and offer various cleaning features. It would be wise to seek advice from your local pool dealer and from other pool owners in your area to deter-

> If dirt accumulation in the pool is light, an alternative to vacuuming is to brush the walls of the pool the day before you intend to vacuum. The brushed dirt will settle on the pool bottom, and you may be able to simply brush the dirt into the main drain while the filter system is on.

Illustration by Wanda Harper

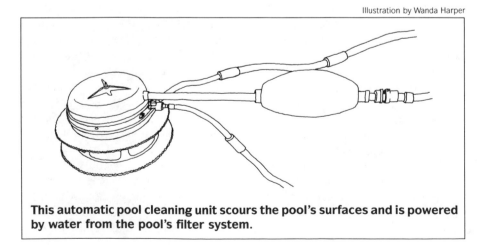

This automatic pool cleaning unit scours the pool's surfaces and is powered by water from the pool's filter system.

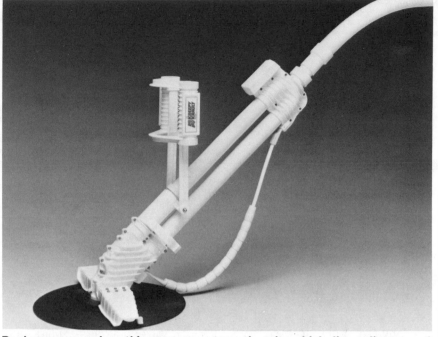

Pool sweeps, such as this one, are automatic units which direct dirt toward the main drain where it is trapped by the filter system.

If the water pressure is too low, the vacuum unit will tend to rise up from the bottom; conversely, if the pressure is too high it can cause the vacuum head to bounce off the bottom or move too fast to pick up dirt.

mine what would be appropriate to your needs.

Everything from an octopus-type automatic cleaner to one with its own filter system is available, and as with other pool components, there are some things to take into consideration. There are models that require the addition of a booster pump for correct operation. This adds to the energy cost and expense of the system. Many automatic cleaners are designed to operate with a pool cover in place. This may or may not be important to you. Some models are designed to operate as sweeps that direct dirt towards the main drain where it is trapped by the pool filter system. Others vacuum dirt, either to their own built-in collection bag or to the pool filter. Automatic cleaners are operated either by water power or electricity.

It's best to have the dealer who ultimately sells you the unit set it up for you also. For water-propelled units, correct adjustment of operating pressures is essential to ensure that they function properly. Man-

ufacturer's literature specifies the correct hose lengths to be used, the water pressure needed at the head, and adjustments needed to make the unit work effectively under given conditions. If the water pressure is too low, the unit will tend to rise up from the bottom; conversely, if the pressure is too high it can cause the head to bounce off the bottom or move too fast to pick up dirt.

If you install one of the automatic pool cleaners that use water pressure, make sure the pump and filter are in good condition. A weak pump and filter system cannot produce the pressure needed to make the unit work. The pump and related plumbing must also be sized to correctly operate the filter and cleaning systems. One final point: if you have the type of automatic cleaner that climbs pool walls and it begins to have trouble doing so, check the walls for algae growth. Algae can cause the walls to become so slick or slippery that the unit will slide off instead of climb. Clean off the algae before calling in a serviceman or the dealer to fix the climbing problem.

9 • Pool Accessories

The range of pool accessories is wide, and growing wider each year. Your own priorities will decide what, if any, accessories you wish to purchase. These might include: a pool cover, ladder and grab rails, portable automatic pool vacuum cleaners, built-in vacuums and pool sweeps, diving board, underwater lights, automatic chemical dispensers, pool fence, windscreens, time clock, gazebo, floating chairs, and a host of other specialized products. Those accessories that are most popular, or which will save you maintenance time, are discussed here.

As with other products, be wary of cheap pool accessories, ones that cannot easily be serviced, and ones for which parts are not easily available.

Photograph provided by the NSPI. Installation: Central Jersey Pools; Freehold, N.J.

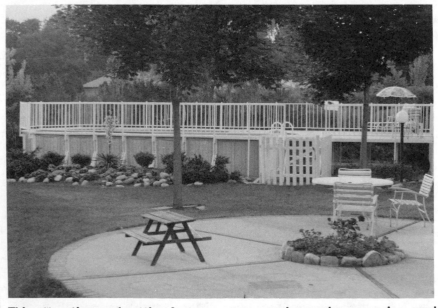

This attractive pool setting features many popular pool accessories: pool fencing, steps, gate, decking, and patio furniture.

Photograph provided by the NSPI. Installation: Central Jersey Pools; Freehold, N.J.

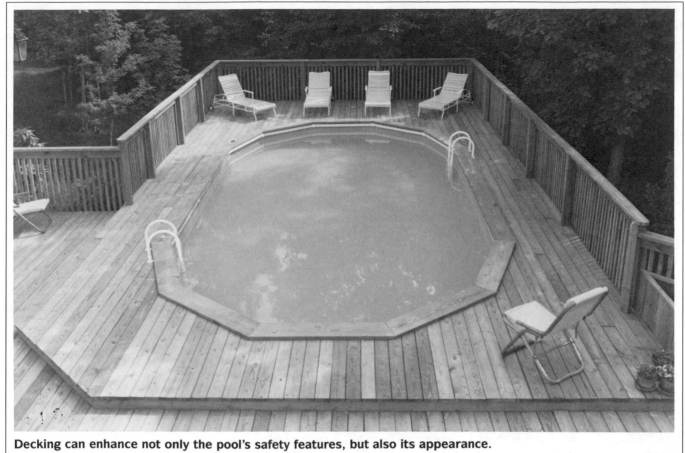

Decking can enhance not only the pool's safety features, but also its appearance.

Pool Decks

Although a pool deck is considered an accessory, it is really more essential than that. A pool without decking made of a suitable material, such as concrete, flagstones, brick, wood, will invite insects, grass clippings, and other debris into the pool. The idea is to provide the pool with an area of protection against insects and debris, as well as a comfortable place to walk, sit, and sunbathe. There are many landscaping books available at libraries and bookstores that discuss pool deck alternatives and ways to turn the pool into an enjoyable and attractive focal point.

Diving Boards

It used to be that diving boards were one of the most popular pool accessories, but adverse publicity emphasizing the large number of crippling accidents associated with the misuse of diving boards has contributed to a decline in their popularity. Safety is the key consideration, as it should also be with slides. The board should be carefully matched to the size and depth of your pool. NSPI does not recommend that pool owners install a diving board. Matching board to pool size is a job for pool builders or contractors only.

If your pool is suitable for installation of a diving board, make certain the board is perfectly aligned with its fulcrum when it is installed. If the board is out of alignment it will twist and become seriously weakened. All anchors that hold the board in place must be firmly attached to the pool deck. If the fastenings that hold the board to its anchors are too tight they can crush the board and become loosened. Choose a board with a nonslip surface and keep the surface in good condition. Most manufacturers recommend that you leave the board in place year-round. Removing the board at the end of each season can damage it more than ice and snow.

Time Clocks and Automatic Controls

Automation has gradually been making advances in pool control systems. Manufacturers have discovered through trial and error that automatic controls and systems must be simple to operate, simple to install, and simple to repair, or pool builders and pool owners won't go for them. They also must remain accurate and reliable over a long period of time and be reasonably priced.

Perhaps the most common automatic pool device is the *time clock*. It is one of the best accessory investments you will ever make, and is standard equipment on most pools today. A time clock can control filtration times, heating, automatic vacuums and sweeps, and even underwater lighting. The most common practice is to connect the time clock to the filtration system so you don't have to remember when to turn it on and—most important as far as energy use is concerned—when to turn it off.

A time clock is basically an electrical switch connected to a built-in, 24-hour clock. Mounted close to the filtration equipment, it is wired into the electrical circuit feeding the pump, and other equipment. The ON and OFF time for the equipment is dialed onto the face of the clock, and at the set time, the filter pump, cleaner, or other equipment turns on automatically, runs for the preset time, then turns itself off. More sophisticated clocks can be installed to control additional functions such as lights or to selectively operate different equipment at different times.

For most pool owners with a family, it will probably be best to run the filter in the early afternoon until about 8 or 10 p.m., depending on how long it takes to "turn over" the total volume of pool water. This will mean that the water has been partially filtered before the kids come home from school, and will ensure that the filter is working while the pool is in use and dirt is being stirred up. Chlorine and other chemicals can then be added in the late evening after swimming is over; the filter will have time to circulate the chemicals completely before shutting down.

It is extremely important to remember that the heater should *never* be switched on (automatically or manually) without water running through it from the pump. For this reason, heaters sold today have a pressure switch, or heater actuator (also known as a fireman's switch), which is connected to the time clock to make sure the heater operates only when the filter pump is in operation. Manufacturers recommend that heaters with an adjustable pressure or fireman's switch should be set to shut off the heater approximately 20 minutes before the filter pump shuts down. This allows residual heat to be carried from the heater to the pool, thereby preventing excessive heat buildup in the exchanger and outlet pipes. It would be wise to check with your pool builder or heater installer to make sure this switch is connected to the time clock and that it works correctly. The majority of heaters today also incorporate a thermostatically controlled switch on the heater so that when the pool water reaches the required temperature, it turns off, regardless of what the pump is doing. If your heater does not have such a control, it is strongly recommended that one be installed to avoid wasting energy.

Also on the market are *automatic chemical feeders* and *digital pool master control panels*, one of which can even be controlled from your car. Radio signals sent to the control unit turn on the pool heater, filtration system, and house or pool

> It is extremely important that the heater *never* be switched on (automatically or manually) without water running through it from the pump.

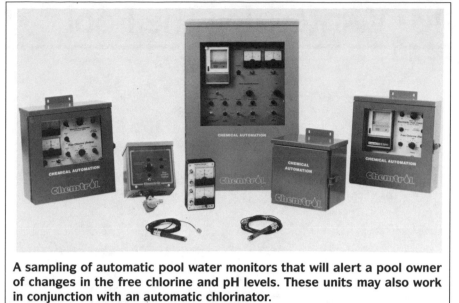

A sampling of automatic pool water monitors that will alert a pool owner of changes in the free chlorine and pH levels. These units may also work in conjunction with an automatic chlorinator.

If you opt for an automatic chlorinator unit that connects to the pool plumbing system, here is a word of caution: the chlorinator must be installed so that the chlorine solution does not flow through the heater.

lights. There are automatic backwash valves and automatic water levellers that sense when the pool level has dropped, and which then refill the pool to the correct level. Automatic chlorine and pH-level controllers have been available in the commercial and public pool market for some time, but only recently have they become available for the residential pool market.

Automatic chlorinators are units that feed chlorine into the pool. They range from simple baskets that hold chlorine in tablet form to units that manufacture their own chlorine from salt dissolved in the pool water and then dispense it into the pool. From the beginning there has been considerable controversy over the effectiveness of automatic chlorinators. These units do not monitor the chlorine or pH levels, as do automatic control units, and therefore the chlorine and pH levels can fluctuate widely if you don't also regularly test the water. Correct professional installation and regular maintenance are essential for automatic chlorinators. Again, investigate the wide variety of units available through local pool supply dealers and seek their advice, as well as that of others who have had experience with such units. If you find from other pool owners that they end up constantly adjusting the chlorinator, it may be simpler and cheaper to do the job manually.

If you opt for an automatic chlorinator unit that connects to the pool plumbing system, here is a word of caution: the chlorinator must be installed so that the chlorine solution does not flow through the heater. If it does, severe corrosion problems can occur. The chlorinator should be installed downstream from the heater. If at all possible, the chlorinator should also be positioned lower than the heater outlet fitting to prevent the chlorine solution from leaking back into the heater. Make sure the chlorinator does not operate without the filter pump running. Check that the chlorinator has an anti-siphoning device to prevent chlorine from siphoning into the heater when the heater outlet pipe drains after the pump is shut off.

Certainly there are many other optional pool accessories. Gather and review product materials at a pool supply dealer, talk with other pool owners, and then decide which accessories are appropriate to your needs and your budget.

10 • Winterizing the Pool

During off-season months when there is little or no swimming your pool will require less maintenance, but still some looking after. In cold climates a pool winterizing routine is essential. It may seem odd to discuss winterizing your pool before a discussion about opening it up for the season, but the ease with which your pool can be readied for summer is greatly dependent on the care exercised in the off-season months.

Whether you live in a mild-winter climate or a cold-winter one, draining the pool for the winter is a poor practice. The National Spa & Pool Institute strongly advises against it. In colder areas the moisture in the ground freezes, which causes tremendous pressure to be exerted against the sides of the pool. If the pool is empty, the pressure can—and often does—buckle or cave in the sides of the pool. The hydrostatic and ice pressure in the ground can also heave the entire pool out of the ground. Some pool owners believe it best to lower the pool level by 2 or 3 feet in the winter, or leave sufficient water in the pool so that it won't be "floated" out of the ground by hydrostatic pressure in the soil. But draining the pool to a considerable extent isn't a good idea. Wet or frozen soil exerts the most pressure against the *top* of the pool walls, and can buckle them or create cracks that will result in expensive repairs unless there is sufficient water in the pool to prevent this.

If you live in an area where the water left in the pool will freeze, be aware that water expands when frozen and that you need to lower the water level enough to allow for expansion. Too much water in the pool will freeze and expand above the pool ground level, which can create pressure against the inside of the pool walls; too little water can create buckling from the pressure of the frozen ground. The trick is to find the happy medium. Don't forget that weather will deposit additional water from rain, snow, and melted ice, and this can raise the pool level quite a bit. Ask friends and neighbors with pools how much pool water they drain off in preparation for winter.

Considering the initial investment you've made in your pool, it would be wise to let a reputable pool service company or your pool builder winterize the pool—at least for the first winter after it's installed. You can then observe the procedure and next winter do it yourself, if you

> Wet or frozen soil exerts the most pressure against the *top* of the pool walls, and can buckle them or create cracks that will result in expensive repairs unless there is sufficient water in the pool to prevent this.

> *Never* use automobile antifreeze — it contains additives that can stain and damage the pool.

want. A reputable company will stand behind their winterizing work. And that is what you want, because if winterizing is not correctly done in a cold climate it can result in thousands of dollars of repair work the following spring. Read the service contract carefully and ask questions. Most companies will not assume responsibility for staining over the winter months, damage to the pool caused by unusual weather conditions, or vandalism. A winterization program will normally include vacuuming the pool, draining and plugging lines, protecting the skimmer box, draining and lubricating the pump, draining the filter, lubricating the heater, and shutting off gas or fuel/electrical lines.

Each company or builder has developed its own winterization procedures, often based on long-term local experience. Ask their advice if you want to do the job yourself. Some service companies in the Midwest and Northeast remove the pool pump for service and storage over the winter. That way, the customer doesn't have to worry about the pump freezing during the winter. Most service companies in colder climates also drain the water from all the lines when winterizing. The lines are blown free of water, plugged, and a special pool antifreeze solution is put in the lines. During this operation, of course, the water level in the pool is usually drained below the level of the pool return lines so it is possible to check that the lines are really clear of water, then the pool is refilled. The skimmer must also be plugged and an empty plastic bottle or piece of wood put in the skimmer to absorb the expansion of any water that gets into the skimmer and freezes. An air compressor or air blower is used to blow the lines dry. The blower is usually connected to the line right at the filter pump.

There is a difference of opinion among professionals as to whether it's better to plug the lines first, then add pool antifreeze, or to add antifreeze and then plug the lines. If added before plugging the lines, the pool antifreeze can be seen coming out of the lines, and you can be sure they are protected. Both suction and return lines must be blown out and plugged. *Never* use automobile antifreeze — it contains additives that can stain and damage the pool.

The safest thing to do with pumps, including the pump in an automatic cleaner, is to remove and store them where there is no danger of freezing. If not, the pump must be thoroughly winterized by removing all moisture. Refer to the manufacturer's instructions on how to drain the pump. Another way to protect the pump is to wrap a heating coil around it, but if there is a power outage the pump could freeze within 1 hour if water is trapped inside.

The filter, valves, and lines to gauges should also be drained. It is often recommended that DE filters be backwashed and the elements removed to allow them to drain and thoroughly dry before replacing. Lights should be removed from their niches in climates where heavy freezing creates enough ice to damage them.

The gas valve on the heater should be turned off. Also turn off the gas valve at the other end of the line, near the meter, if there is one. If the pilot light must be left on for some reason, turn the gas valve to PILOT ONLY position. Drain the header in the heater as specified in the owner's manual. Check the manufacturer's instructions: some recommend draining the pressure switch in the heater, but others do not.

The final step is to bring the water to the correct level for your area, adjust the pH level, and add a stabilizer to prevent the pH level from dropping over the winter months. Some pool service companies recommend superchlorinating the pool at this point, others don't because bacteria growth slows down considerably in cold water. The danger of adding chlorine to a cold pool is that it tends to sink to the floor and can bleach colored vinyl liners. Some pool services recommend using a lithium-based chlorine for superchlorinating during winterization because it is completely soluble and won't attack liner surfaces or pipes. The addition of an algaecide to control algae growth is vital.

In addition to the above tasks, all electrical wires to the equipment should be disconnected at the fuse or breaker box.

Another problem in winterization is the main drain at the bottom of the pool. The only safe way to protect it against freezing is to drain the pool completely, fill the main drain with pool antifreeze and plug it, then refill the pool. However, many pool service companies can avoid this by blowing a bubble of air into the main drain. This works well as long as the main drain doesn't "burp" and lose its protective bubble of air. In most areas of the country, the frost line will not reach down far enough to cause any problems. But again, seek advice from a knowledgeable local expert because in some regions the frost line penetrates to such a depth that special precautions must be taken.

Covering the Pool

During the months when the pool is not in use it is highly recommended that the pool be covered with a winter cover. Leaves, debris, and dirt that have been washed and blown into the pool over the winter can present a huge cleanup job in the spring, and some plaster pools may even have to be acid-washed before they can be used. A cover will keep out dirt and debris, considerably reducing the need for chemicals, and will block out sunlight minimizing the formation of algae.

Winter covers also prevent damage to pool surfaces. In a vinyl-liner pool there is the danger that wind can push slushy or frozen pool water against the walls, which can puncture the liner if the ice is jagged or sharp. Even with plastered concrete pools, ice can chip the surface. A winter cover will virtually eliminate this problem.

To minimize damage from expanding ice on the pool surface, there are a number of devices available from pool supply stores, including air bags, balloons, and foam sheets. These also help to keep the cover from sagging.

Pool covers should be large enough to overlap the pool edges by at least 2 to 3 feet. Many owners float a large beach ball in the water to help support the cover. Rain and melted snow will accumulate on the cover, however, and should be siphoned off regularly with a garden hose, or any small pump. Pool covers that are put on and taken off manually must be held down securely around the sides of the pool. The best method consists of an anchoring system set flush into the deck. Using water bags is less expensive. Some covers are designed with integral bags; less expensive covers have ties to secure separate water bags. A check with pool owners reveals that those with attached bags seem to have less problems. Lightweight mesh-type covers are gaining in popularity. Being lightweight, they are easier to put on and take off. The mesh is extremely fine, so only minute particles enter the water. They do let sunlight into the pool, though, so it is necessary to test the water periodically and adjust the chlorine level.

Winter-type pool covers are large and heavy, so they require at least two or three people to handle them. The usual way to put on this type of cover is to set it at one end of the pool and secure the end. Then two people each take a free end and pull it lengthwise across the pool. While doing this, be careful not to drop the cover into the pool. Getting it

The danger of adding chlorine to a cold pool is that it tends to sink to the floor and can bleach colored vinyl liners.

When closing the pool for the winter, all electrical wires to the equipment should be disconnected at the fuse or breaker box.

Illustration by Chrysalis Design Group

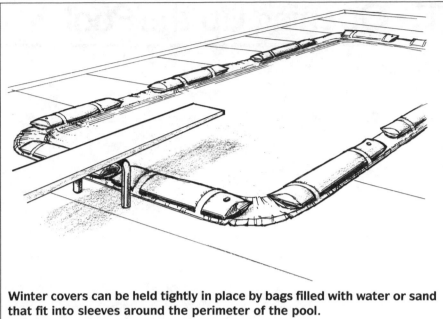

Winter covers can be held tightly in place by bags filled with water or sand that fit into sleeves around the perimeter of the pool.

out again can be quite a job. When the cover is in place, tie it down or secure it with water or sand bags. Leave the water bags only two-thirds full to allow room for ice expansion.

Mild Climate Off-Season Care

In milder climates, where there is no risk of freezing, pool care is simply a continuation of normal season pool care, but there is less of it. With swimming at a minimum, there is not as much need for chemical sanitizing and filtration. Colder temperatures and reduced swimming greatly cut down on the growth of algae or bacteria. You may have some problem with leaves in the fall and with flower blossoms in the early spring, but the installation of a pool cover will do away with this problem.

Turn off the pool heater—following manufacturer's directions—when there is not as much need for it. Some recommend that the pilot light be left on to prevent moisture from collecting in the lines. The filtering cycle can usually be cut in half. Check water balance (pH, calcium, hardness, and chlorine residual) once a week, and adjust to appropriate levels. Also check and clean out the skimmer box and pump leaf strainer faithfully. If the pool is uncovered, you should still vacuum and brush the walls when they begin to look dirty. This will reduce the chances of staining.

Wherever you live, the routine or preparation for the winter months is an essential part of proper pool maintenance.

11 • Opening Up the Pool

If your pool has been sufficiently winterized (in milder climates that means a regular but reduced maintenance schedule) then opening it for the swimming season should be relatively easy. Most of the work involves cleaning. Again, you can opt to have a pool service company do the work, or you can do it yourself. In cold climates where full winterization by a pool service company is necessary (pumps and other equipment have been shut down and lines blocked), it may be easier and wiser to have the same company reopen the pool for you.

The first task, in any case, is to pump or siphon any water that has accumulated on the pool cover, and remove any dirt, leaves, and other debris. Once the cover is clean, you can safely remove it. If, by chance, the cover should drop into the pool while it is being removed, at least you won't be dumping in a winter's accumulation of dirt. When it comes to removing a winter cover, the more people you have to help, the better. It will require at least two people for a medium-size pool. When the cover is off, lay it out on the ground and scrub it with a stiff broom and detergent. Rinse the cover and let it dry thoroughly before storing it in a clean, dry place away from the sun. Pool supply stores sell a special talcum powder that helps prevent mildew problems on winter covers.

If the lines had been blown out and filled with pool antifreeze, they must be unblocked and the antifreeze removed. Be careful not to let the antifreeze run into the pool. Lower the water level until the blocked lines are exposed, then remove the plugs and drain the pool antifreeze into a bucket. Blowing or flushing the lines is recommended to remove all the antifreeze. This is a good time to check the tile coping around the pool for any damage or scale formation, and to remove any water stains before refilling the pool.

If your pool was empty over the winter months, the first job is to sweep it out and inspect the walls and bottom for cracks in concrete or fiberglass pools, or tears in the vinyl liner. These will need to be repaired before the pool is filled. When checking the walls and bottom, look for depressions or similar signs of structural damage. If it appears that there has been structural damage, call in a pool repair company. They will give you a report on the damage and an estimate. You can then decide what to do about it. In vinyl-

Be careful not to let the antifreeze run into the pool.

> Don't wait a few days before testing the water and bringing it into balance — by that time, bacteria and algae may be flourishing and will be harder to remove.

liner pools with a sand foundation beneath the liner, "washouts" sometimes occur from exceptionally heavy rains or spring thaw. Poor drainage can also cause washouts. These show as a depression in the bottom of the pool. Minor washouts can be left alone, but if it's a major washout, the liner may be resting on stones or rocks, and would therefore be susceptible to puncture. In this case, the liner must be removed and the washout repaired. Fortunately, minor tears in vinyl can be repaired without removing the liner, even while the pool is full of water. Repair kits can be obtained from a local pool supply dealer.

If the pump has been removed, reinstall it. Check and reconnect the wiring and pipes. Make sure all the fittings are clean and tight, and replace any drainage plugs, valves, and pressure gauges that were removed for the winter. Check the filter for cracks in the casing, and if you have a sand filter, check for mudballs and remove them. DE filters require a slurry of diatomaceous earth and water circulated through the filter to coat the screens before the filter is put into service. Follow the instructions from the manufacturer. The usual recommendation is 2 ounces of diatomaceous earth for each square foot of surface area. The recommendation is stamped on the manufacturer's plate on the filter. When first starting the filter after a long period of disuse, put the filter in the backwash mode. That way, any dirt in the lines will be flushed into the wasteline rather than dumped into the pool.

Fill the pump to the correct level and make sure the skimmer weir (flap) is operating correctly and in the right position. With the pump reconnected, open up the main drain and skimmer valves. Prime the pump and observe the valves as the pump and filter start up. Over the winter, packings and gaskets within valves probably will have dried out if not in use. They may leak for a time, but normally will stop leaking once normal use has resumed. If they still leak, the valves probably require new gaskets or may have a structural defect, in which case they will have to be replaced. Turn off the power until a service person has made the needed repairs or adjustments.

Prime the pump by filling the leaf strainer with water. Make sure the valves between the pump and filter are open. A new pump should start pumping water almost immediately. If this is not the case, turn off the motor, remove the strainer cover and check the impeller — it may be clogged or stuck. On some pumps it is possible to loosen a jammed impeller by turning it manually.

Once the pump is running, check the system for leaks, open valves, and split pipes. If everything seems to be okay, switch the filter valve to the FILTER position to begin filtration of the pool.

At first, the water may appear cloudy. It will take some time for the filter to clean the water. When the water is relatively clear, test and adjust the water balance and chlorine levels. Most professionals recommend superchlorination when opening up the pool for two reasons: one is to get rid of any bacteria or algae formations; the other is to thoroughly cleanse the water. The super dose of chlorine "burns up" suspended dirt in the water. If there are obvious signs of algae growth, add an algaecide. Don't wait a few days before testing the water and bringing it into balance — by that time, bacteria and algae may be flourishing and will be harder to remove. It may be necessary to run the filter almost continuously for the first 4 or 5 days to clear the water so it can be properly balanced. After that, you can resume routine water treatment, a normal filtration cycle, and any other maintenance procedures you follow.

12 • Pool Face-Lifts

A well-constructed pool will last many years before it deteriorates to such a point that it requires a face-lift. But accidents do happen—pool water is inadvertently allowed to remain out of balance, which can stain or mar the finish; sometimes the ground shifts and cracks appear in walls or floor; or time and use take their toll on pool surfaces.

With plaster-finished pools, the most common face-lift treatment is to have it professionally acid-washed to remove 'stains. Such pools can also be patched, replastered, painted, or fiberglassed. Painted concrete pools can be similarly upgraded and painted with a waterproof coating or fiberglassed.

Fiberglass pools can be revitalized with a new paint coating. Sunlight and chemicals can produce fading, staining, or even blistering over a long period of time, but a new paint job can restore the pool to its former glory for many more years of service.

Vinyl-liner pools cannot, of course, be rejuvenated with paint. Holes in the liner can be repaired, but once a liner has faded, the only way to bring back that new pool appearance is to replace the liner. These days, a new vinyl liner need not be any more expensive than a paint job—in some cases, less. Basic information on pool renovation follows, arranged under the type of pool to be renovated, but first some general comments on pool coatings.

Coatings

Pool paint—or pool coatings, as they are called in the trade—are specifically designed for pool use. Ordinary oil-based or acrylic paints cannot withstand the constant immersion in chemically active pool water. Buy the best pool coating you can afford—it is false economy to buy cheap pool paint.

The two most widely used pool coatings today are rubber-based and epoxy. *Natural chlorinated rubber* has proven itself as a pool coating over many years. Advantages include ease of preparation, excellent water resistance, strong adhesion, and a smooth, hard finish that is resistant to pool chemicals. Once a pool has been properly painted with a chlorinated rubber coating it is easy to repaint with the same type of coating. The solvent in the new coat softens and penetrates the old coat so that the two coats become

After choosing a good-quality paint that is compatible with the pool surface to be painted, the most important step is surface preparation.

A successful paint job requires that the pool surfaces be thoroughly cleaned to remove all traces of body oils, grease, or dirt.

as one. A chlorinated rubber coating should provide 3 or more years of service life.

Epoxy pool coatings offer a smooth, tilelike finish, and excellent chemical, abrasion, and algae resistance, but they do require skill in application. In recent years, new formulations of epoxy paints, in combination with special primers, have greatly improved the resistance of these coatings to chalking and delamination, which were problems with earlier epoxy paints. These new epoxy coatings can be applied to concrete, plaster, steel, or aluminum pools. They are, of course, the only type of coating to use on fiberglass pools, where they provide excellent bonding between the fiberglass and epoxy coating. The service life of epoxy coatings is generally 4 to 6 years.

Preparation and Application

After choosing a good-quality paint that is compatible with the pool surface to be painted, the most important step is surface preparation. The second most important step is to pay careful attention to the paint manufacturer's application instructions. Reputable pool coatings manufacturers provide detailed technical bulletins and other support literature for their products. The instructions that follow are necessarily of a general nature, and the manufacturer's instructions may vary, depending on the type of coating and primers used.

The majority of pool paint failures are caused by improper surface preparation. A successful paint job requires that the pool surfaces be thoroughly cleaned to remove all traces of body oils, grease, or dirt. The surfaces must then be roughened or etched so the new paint will penetrate and adhere to it.

Fiberglass pools. Clean the fiberglass pool surfaces with an abrasive household cleanser or a TSP

(trisodium phosphate) solution, then hose off and allow to dry. Roughen the surface with a fine or medium-grit sandpaper. Apply a coat of primer and one or two coats of epoxy paint.

Previously painted pools. If the pool has been previously painted and if 20 percent or less of the pool surface is peeling or scaling, you can touch up the old coating. Remove all loose or scaling paint by light sanding, wash with a TSP compound, then hose off.

To provide maximum adhesion of the new paint, the old finish should be etched, whether you are touching up or completely repainting the pool. Etch the surface with a 10 to 20 percent solution of muriatic or hydrochloric acid (it is 10 to 20 percent acid and 80 to 90 percent water). This will remove calcium and salt formations that have built up over a period of time. When acid-washing, do not allow the acid solution to dry on the surface. Scrub one section with a long-handled brush, then flush it with fresh water before going on to the next section. If allowed to dry, the acid creates crystal formations that can cause the paint to blister later on.

If more than 20 percent of the pool surface coating is peeling or scaling, all the old paint will have to be removed by sandblasting or high-powered water blasting. Blasting off old paint is a big job; if it is professionally removed, you could probably do the repainting yourself by following the guidelines in this chapter. But don't attempt to sandblast or water blast without the help or advice of a pool service professional.

Plaster and concrete pools. Painting bare concrete or plaster-finished pools requires that the surface be completely clean and free of grease, oils, and dirt, and that the surface be etched or sandblasted. For maximum adhesion, concrete or plaster surfaces should have the appearance and feel of fine-grade sandpaper. Remember, acid-etching alone will not remove grease or oil — for that you need a detergent or TSP solution.

Fine, hairline cracks in concrete or plaster that do not penetrate the pool shell will normally fill in adequately when new paint is applied. Check for cracks *before* emptying the pool. If a piece of tissue paper held near the crack is sucked into it, the pool has a leak that must be repaired before painting. (See the following chapter on pool repairs.) Such cracks will not only allow pool water to drain away (expensive and damaging), but will allow moisture from the ground around the pool to penetrate the pool shell and cause blistering and delamination of the paint.

A word of warning about acid-etching or acid-washing pool surfaces. Muriatic or hydrochloric acid produce dangerous fumes. Make sure there is adequate ventilation — if there is not a vigorous breeze, use an electric fan in the pool to blow away acid fumes. Wear a safety mask, safety glasses, rubber gloves, and an apron. Even pool repair professionals have been overcome by fumes when acid-washing a pool, so you might consider the potential risks against the cost of employing an expert. If you decide to do this work yourself, make sure the brush handle is long enough so that you don't get splashed. When mixing acid, always pour the acid into the water. *Never pour water into the acid* — it will explode in your face.

Paint Compatibility

If you plan to repaint a previously painted pool, it is vital to use a paint that is compatible with the old paint. If you know the brand and type of old paint, it makes things that much easier — you can check with a paint manufacturer or pool supply retailer. Compatibility does not mean paint of the same brand — it means that the chemical composition of the paint is compatible.

If you plan to paint over a coating of unknown composition, you must test it first for compatibility. To find

---

GENERAL PAINTING TIPS

- Small- to medium-size pools can be painted with a 9-inch roller. Use a 5-gallon bucket with a roller grid that fits it. Excess paint is rolled off on the grid after the roller is dipped in paint. Use paint from a can that is one-quarter to two-thirds full. For larger pools, an airless spray gun is best. If you are going to use a roller, get an adjustable roller handle (adjusts from 14 to 18 inches) and use heavy-duty paint pans. These pans can be dragged along the floor of the pool.
- Always allow plenty of time for drying between coats. Some paints require up to 7 days or more to cure before refilling the pool with water. When the ground around a plastered or concrete pool is saturated with water, such as after heavy rain, the pool must be allowed to "dry out" for 2 to 4 days before painting. Moisture from the soil migrates through the plaster or concrete to evaporate into the air. If painted before the pool is dry, this moisture can cause the paint to blister.

- Paint the pool walls first and floor last. Paint the last floor section near a ladder so you can climb out. Never wear hard-soled shoes when painting — only soft-soled shoes or sneakers.
- Avoid painting in direct sunlight on hot days. Start on the shady side and try to follow the sun around the pool, painting in the shade whenever possible. Hot direct sunlight starts the paint drying from the outside surface inward, sealing in the solvent. As the heat of the sun expands the solvent, blisters can result.
- Areas of the pool that will not air dry, such as the area around the main drain, can be dried using any electric heater with a fan to blow air.
- When using a spray applicator, cover surfaces that will not be painted with masking paper or polyethylene cut to size. Drains, outlets, inlets, and underwater lights should be removed before painting and left off until finished. Cover the pool deck with drop cloths.

---

out if an old coating is rubber based, take a small chip of old paint and immerse it in a rubber-based paint solvent. If it softens, the paint is rubber-based. Another way to test paint composition is to apply the new paint to several small test areas and allow it to dry for several hours. It would be wise to do this even when you know the paint brand and type, just in case there has been a mistake or change in paint formulation. If there is any wrinkling, cracking, bleeding, or blistering, the new paint is not compatible with the old coating. You will either have to experiment to find one that is compatible or completely remove the old coating and start from scratch. If there are no obvious changes in the texture of the new paint test patches, don't paint just yet. Wait for another 24 hours, then scratch the test areas with a piece of metal or with your fingernail. If the two paints cannot be separated easily, chances are they are compatible enough to give a satisfactory final finish.

13 • Pool Repairs to do Yourself

Major pool damage caused by earth movement, mudslides, incorrect installation, ice pressure, or washout, can be discouraging, but don't make any drastic decisions (such as turning the pool into a tennis court) until you have estimates from at least three reputable pool builders in your area. If the damage is not catastrophic, you will probably be able to do the repair work yourself.

CRACKS AND LEAKS

Cracks or leaks in concrete, plaster, fiberglass, and vinyl-liner pools should be suspected whenever there is a steady drop in the pool level, particularly in cool weather or when the pool is seldom used. A certain amount of water is lost from normal evaporation, splashing, and filter cleaning, but when water loss is excessive, it could be a leak. All leaks should be repaired as soon as possible, because leaking water can undermine the pool and deck, and even exert enough pressure through soil expansion that the pool shell can be damaged.

In concrete and plaster pools, hairline cracks that are not deep enough to allow water to seep through the shell can be easily filled in with paint, a hydraulic cement mixture, or calking compound available at pool supply stores. One way to tell if the crack is allowing water to escape from the pool is to hold a facial tissue near it—if the tissue is drawn into the crack, you've got a leak that must be repaired. To fill large cracks you must enlarge them with a cold chisel, undercutting the edges so that the old concrete or plaster overhangs the edges of the area to "lock" the patching compound in place (Figure 13.1). Clean the area with a wire brush, removing all loose material and dust, then wet the area to be patched (or follow the procedure in the manufacturer's directions). With some hydraulic cement mortars, the mixture is forced into the damaged area, levelled off, and the area kept wet for anywhere from several hours to as long as 3 days to properly cure and harden.

If there are no obvious cracks, check around the tile line, fittings, lights and any bolt-through anchors below the waterline. Again hold a piece of facial tissue near the suspected leak. Or use an eyedropper with a visible food coloring—squeeze a few drops into the water near the suspected leak. If the coloring is sucked into the crack or suspected leaking area you're losing water through the pool surface. To repair leaks around lights or fittings, you'll have to drain the pool below the level of the fitting and either calk or patch the area, depending on the nature of the damage. Make sure the electricity is turned off before tackling any work near pool light fixtures.

Repairs to vinyl. Repairing a tear or leak in a vinyl-liner pool is a relatively simple task. You can buy vinyl patching kits from a pool dealer or supplier—some kits can be used underwater so you don't have to drain the pool. If you can't find a kit, then get a sheet of vinyl that matches the liner of your pool. Cut a piece that overlaps the tear by at least 1 inch. Clean the liner surface with a household cleanser. The patching kit should include glue, but if not buy a brand for vinyl liner repairs at a pool supply store. Paint both the patch and the pool liner with the glue. Smooth the patch firmly in place. The solvent in the glue will cause the two pieces of vinyl to dissolve, then harden into a fusion bond equal in strength to the rest of the liner.

Repairs to fiberglass. If a crack or leak occurs in a fiberglass pool shell, the pool must be drained down to the crack and the material relaminated. Generally speaking, this is work for a pool repair company. If you want to tackle it yourself, be sure to consult someone who has done this kind of repair, and wear proper protective clothing: mask, strong gloves, and goggles. You will have to grind down the top layer of gelcoat to expose the fiberglass laminate beneath, otherwise the patch will pop out or the cracking

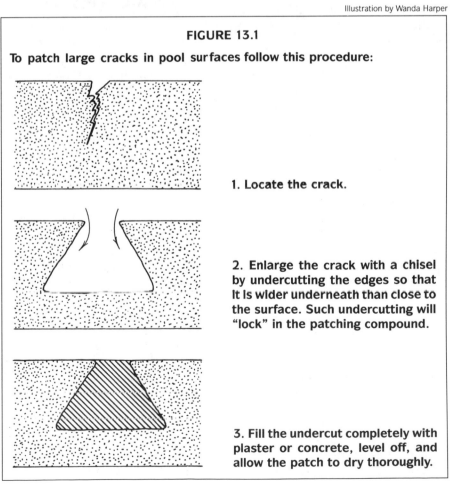

Illustration by Wanda Harper

FIGURE 13.1

To patch large cracks in pool surfaces follow this procedure:

1. Locate the crack.

2. Enlarge the crack with a chisel by undercutting the edges so that it is wider underneath than close to the surface. Such undercutting will "lock" in the patching compound.

3. Fill the undercut completely with plaster or concrete, level off, and allow the patch to dry thoroughly.

will continue. You need to grind away the area for several inches past the farthest extension of the crack. If the crack is a "leaker" — it extends down through the fiberglass mat layers so that water is leaking from the pool — you will have to grind the area down then lay up several layers of fiberglass mat before putting the top gelcoat on. Suppliers of fiberglass mat and gelcoats can be found in the Yellow Pages.

Color matching the repair patch to the rest of the pool requires care and a good eye for color. Manufacturers and distributors supply gelcoat color matched to certain standard colors, but often the color of the pool has faded somewhat from its original appearance. In this case you need to use a universal light toner for adjusting the gelcoat to a lighter shade. To adjust the gelcoat to a darker shade, you add a dark toner. One technique is to place a measured amount (30 to 60 grams) of the gelcoat in a cup, add the toner in very small increments, stirring with a wooden spatula or the stick from a Popsicle. Once an acceptable color match is obtained, apply the gelcoat according to the manufacturer's directions.

Fiberglass mats are saturated with resin mixed with approximately 2 percent catalyst (follow manufacturer's instructions exactly), then placed over the damaged area one at a time. Use a brush or roller to eliminate all air bubbles and loose spots. Leave the mats to cure for about 2 hours. Then apply the top gelcoat according to instructions. Usually this involves thickening the gelcoat mix until the gelcoat putty is creamy on the surface. The catalyst is added and the mixture quickly applied with a flexible spatula or piece of flexible plastic. You can speed up curing with a heat gun or hair dryer, but don't let it get too hot or it will cure too rapidly and crack. Once the patch is cured it should be sanded. Pool repair professionals generally use a 220- or 230-grit wet-or-dry sandpaper, progressing to a 400- to 600-grit paper. Then the area is buffed with a cotton buffing pad covered with jeweler's rouge or a similar compound, until you get a high gloss. The final step is to wax the patched area. When done right, such repairs are practically invisible to the eye.

If a concrete shell pool is badly cracked and shifted, it may be necessary to pour/spray a new 3- or 4-inch reinforced concrete shell inside the old shell. The surface of the old shell will have to be sandblasted and then etched with acid to provide a good bond. This is *definitely* a job for a pool repair company. The exact cause for the cracking and shifting must be identified and remedied before the new shell is poured, or the same thing could happen again.

Leaking Below-Ground Lines

A leak in an underground water line can be one of the most frustrating problems encountered — first to find the leak, next to repair it. Constant and above-normal water loss is the sign of a leak. To determine whether the leak is from the pool shell or from the water lines, plug the wall inlets and skimmer box. If the pool stops losing water after the filter lines have been plugged, it is a safe bet that the leak is not in the pool shell but in one of the lines to and from the filter. An obvious indicator of a leaking line is a wet spot or depression in the ground above the filter lines. Air bubbles in the return waterline from the filter to the pool, indicates the pump is sucking air and could mean there is a leak in the skimmer or intake line. Close off each line in succession. If the bubbles in the return line cease when you close the skimmer valve, chances are the leak is in that line.

Once you've identified the leaking line, the problem now is how to fix the leak. In most cases it is far easier to install a new line and abandon

If a concrete shell pool is badly cracked and shifted, it will have to be sandblasted and then etched with acid to provide a good bond. This is *definitely* a job for a pool repair company.

the old one, particularly if it means digging up the pool decking or a concrete patio to repair the damaged line. Call in a service company and have them repair or replace the leaking pipe. If you have determined the source of the leak, you will have saved them time, and saved yourself some money.

Replacing a Vinyl Liner

One of the advantages of a vinyl-liner pool is that the liner can be replaced. Most liners should last up to 10 years. After that, they tend to become brittle, faded, and weak from chemicals and sunlight. A liner must be cut to fit your pool exactly. If the manufacturer of your pool is no longer in business or cannot be found, you can obtain a custom-made liner from any number of liner fabricators that can be located in the Yellow Pages or through the NSPI.

It would be smart to allow the fabricator to measure the pool—if you measure it and make a mistake, the fabricator cannot be held responsible. If you cannot get a fabricator to come to your pool, most of them use standard liner order forms that detail all the measurements needed and how to take them.

Basically, a fabricator needs a plan view (top view) of the pool, as well as side and end views. If the pool has curved corners, he needs to know the corner radii. End and side view dimensions are needed for every change in plane. Measurements should be made on horizontal and vertical planes and not along angles, such as the slope into the deep end. Measurements are, of course, much easier to take if there is no water in the pool. To measure depth in the center of the pool, use masonry twine pulled taut across the pool as a guideline.

Two people can install a vinyl liner, but it is better to have four people. Clean and inspect the pool before installing the new liner. Wipe down the panels to remove dirt. If the pool has a sand bottom, make sure the sand is smooth and even with no protruding rocks or debris. If you are going to install a new liner in cool weather, store the liner in a heated room for a day or two. This will make it easier to handle and smooth out any wrinkles caused by packing.

Set the folded liner at one end of the pool so that you can unroll it as you walk down the length of the pool. If there are only two of you, anchor one end with a heavy board or rocks. If four people are available, station one at each corner. While two people walk their corners of the liner toward the opposite end of the pool, unfolding it as they go, the other two hold their two corners stationary. The idea is to finish with the liner correctly suspended above the sand or concrete bottom with all sections in their correct positions.

The liner is installed into the coping lip, starting with the corners. Each corner has a mark that must fit exactly with the corners of the pool. When the corners are correctly fitted, insert the rest of the liner bead (thick edge) into the coping groove. You'll probably have to tug the liner at a number of points to get it into correct position. Take a heavy fold of material with both hands and pull in short tugs. The liner will take a lot of stress without damage. Once the liner is in place and secured all around by the coping, remove the air between the liner and wall panels. To prevent air leaks, use tape to close off the skimmer and any wall fittings, then insert a vacuum hose between the liner and walls to a point about 18 inches below the top of the pool walls. As the vacuum hose sucks the air out, work the liner with your hands to remove all the wrinkles. Any wrinkles left in the liner will be there permanently when the pool is filled with water. It should take about 15 or 20 minutes to fully collapse the liner against the pool wall.

Keep the vacuum hose going while you fill the pool until there is about 6 inches of water in the shallow end. You can then remove the vacuum hose and reinsert the bead of the liner back into the coping lip. And don't forget to untape the skimmer and fittings.

Fiberglassing Pools

Concrete pools with leaks or structural problems can often be renovated by lining the pool with fiberglass. If the pool has been painted with a rubber-based paint, this must be removed first. If you've had experience with fiberglassing techniques, you could undertake the job yourself, preferably with the help of some friends. Generally, though, it would be best to let a reputable pool repair company do the fiberglassing. Choose a company with experience in this type of work. The task of fiberglassing is not made any easier by the toxic, quick-setting solvents and resins that must be used (these often set within 15 minutes or less after mixing), and handling of the fiberglass mats with their sharp, irritating fibers.

The procedure followed by the service company will be to etch the walls of the pool with a mild solution of acid and water. When the solution has been rinsed clean and the walls are dry, resin-soaked fiberglass mats are applied to the walls, overlapping all seams. The mats are smoothed with a roller to eliminate all air bubbles and to evenly distribute the resin. The layer of fiberglass mats is allowed to cure, then the rough spots are ground down with a power sander. The final result should not be smooth—the surface texture should resemble that of an orange peel. Fiberglass resin is then applied and allowed to set, then the final gelcoat (with color mixed in) is applied. Correctly done, fiberglassing can be an excellent solution to a problem pool, the smooth finish will resist dirt and algae buildup, and will not affect water pH levels.

14 • Pool Safety

Every pool owner should have a copy of *The Sensible Way to Enjoy Your Pool*, a safety guide available from the National Spa & Pool Institute for a small fee. Their address can be found on page 1. It covers swimming, safe use of diving boards and pool slides, exercise, safety equipment, and tips for poolside entertaining. The thing to remember is that as a pool owner, you are ultimately responsible and liable for the safety of everyone using your pool.

Supervision is the key to pool safety. One person should be designated to enforce *pool rules*. These rules can be drawn up from booklets such as the NSPI booklet mentioned above or those available from the YMCA and American Red Cross. The rules should cover safe use of diving boards, slides, games, and safe handling of chemicals. When you've drawn up a list of pool rules post them in plain sight near the pool, and be sure that people know and follow them. It is particularly important to educate young children about safety precautions; teach them what to do in case of emergency even if they are not allowed to use the pool without adult supervision. Have a meeting with regulars users of your pool every year to review the rules you have established. As a general rule, if you're not comfortable with someone's swimming ability, ask them stay in shallow water and keep an eye them. Do not allow anyone to swim alone. And discourage anyone from swimming who is tired or chilled, those who have just eaten, or who have taken drugs or alcohol.

In addition to a broad set of rules that apply to your pool and pool area, please be aware of some other safety considerations that follow.

Diving and sliding. Diving or sliding into a pool poses a serious risk to those unfamiliar with the dangers. Don't allow horseplay around diving boards and slides. Serious spinal injuries can occur, even at slow speeds, if the diver's head strikes firmly against the pool bottom or side. Research shows that water alone will not slow you down sufficiently—you must take precautions by steering up with your hands. As you enter the water, extend your arms over your head aimed upward. Hold your head up and arch your back so your whole body will steer upward, away from the bottom. Most headfirst accidents happen in shallow water—don't dive or slide headfirst into the shallow end of the pool. Alcohol and drugs have also been found to play a major role in serious diving and sliding accidents.

Diving accidents in lakes, streams, and pools cause hundreds of serious spinal cord injuries annually in this country. The National Swimming Pool Foundation (an educational and research foundation) in cooperation with the NSPI sponsored an 8-year research program on diving safety. The NSPI produced a booklet based on the results of this research, "Knowing How to Dive is as Important as Learning How to Swim." Here are some basic diving tips:

- When you dive, steer up immediately after entering the water. Keep your hands tipped up, your head back, and your back arched. In other words, *don't dive too deep*.
- Always keep your hands in front of your head.
- Plan your dive path into the water before you dive.
- Don't dive into any unknown waters; make sure there are no submerged or floating obstacles.
- No back dives or running dives should be allowed.
- Do not dive across the narrow part of a pool.
- Do not add diving equipment to pools that are not designed for diving.

Entertaining. It can be a lot of fun to entertain people at poolside, but remember to keep food and drinks away from the pool to avoid getting debris in the water. Use unbreakable dishes and beverage containers. Broken glass is invisible in water and difficult to get out of the pool equipment. Keep all eating and cooking utensils and electrical appliances a safe distance from the pool and make sure you have a ground fault circuit interrupter (GFCI) on any appliance that is at poolside. Be sure you know the safe maximum capacity of your pool, and do not

allow it be exceeded. You are responsible for knowing how many people are in your pool, and then keeping an eye on them.

Whenever practical, people using your pool should first shower with soap and water to wash away common skin bacteria, skin lotions, deodorants, and creams, which can lessen the efficiency of your filter and reduce the effectiveness of the pool disinfectant. People with skin, ear, genital or other body infections, or open sores or wounds, should not be allowed to use the pool—there is a danger of spreading infection to others. When there is a rainstorm or the threat of lightning, keep people out of the pool. They can be electrocuted if lightning strikes the water.

Entertaining at night requires special equipment and attention. Swimming after dark should only be allowed in an area that has floodlights and in a pool that has lights installed under the water surface. If you plan a night pool party, it is good sense and good manners to inform your neighbors, and tell them you will try to keep the noise down. You might even set a time after which swimming must stop out of courtesy to your neighbors.

Safe operation of equipment. The safe operation of equipment around the pool is mainly a matter of common sense: reading, understanding, and following the instructions that come with the equipment. When investigating the source of a problem in your pool system, you should *always* turn off the power *before* you stick your hands, tools, or head into any mechanical or electrical device.

Covers. Always completely remove the pool cover before using the pool to avoid the possibility of someone becoming trapped under it. Remove standing water that accumulates on the cover surface—even a small amount of water can be hazardous to toddlers and pets who may fall onto the cover.

Make sure you have a ground fault circuit interrupter (GFCI) on any appliance that is at poolside.

When investigating the source of a problem in your pool system, you should *always* turn off the power *before* you stick your hands, tools, or head into any mechanical or electrical device.

Decks. Make sure the deck or patio around the pool has a slip-resistant surface and good drainage. Slips and falls represent the largest number of pool accidents. Keep the deck or patio clean and free of debris. Insist that there be no running, pushing, or roughhousing near the pool, and that throwing anyone into the pool is absolutely forbidden.

Accessories and equipment. Check the condition and mounting of all accessories periodically: diving boards, slides, steps, tile, inlets, and light fixtures. If any of these become loose or chipped, immediately discontinue their use until proper repairs can be made.

Fences. Pools attract children, so in most areas of the country a pool fence is mandatory by law to keep children or pets out of the pool when it is not supervised. The gate should have a self-closing and self-latching spring lock, installed well above the reach of toddlers or young children. If you have an above-ground pool, either install a ladder or steps that are removable or that swing up when the pool is not in use. The height of the fence is usually specified in municipal codes and your local pool builder will have these.

Grates and drains. Instruct all swimmers, particularly children, not to stick their fingers or toes in pool

Illustration by Wanda Harper

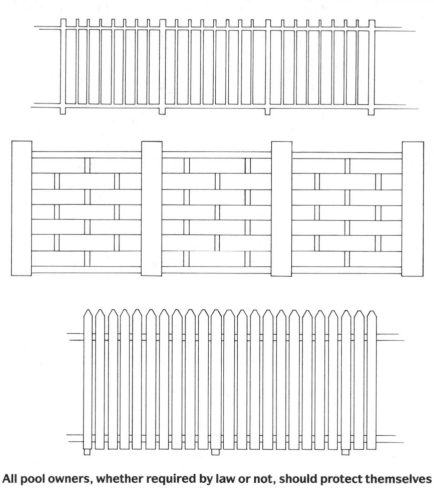

All pool owners, whether required by law or not, should protect themselves and their property by installing a fence (and secure gate) around the pool area. Shown here is a simple banister-type fence for wood or metal, a basketweave fence, and a picket fence.

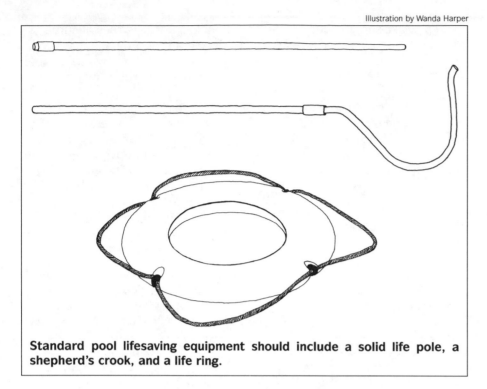

Standard pool lifesaving equipment should include a solid life pole, a shepherd's crook, and a life ring.

fittings, grates, and drains, or put their body against them. The suction can trap and/or injure swimmers. Make sure all of the pool's inlet and outlet fittings, grates, and skimmer and main drain covers are in good repair, and secured in place at all times, except when cleaning. A main drain without a grate in place can exert a pull of approximately 700 pounds—more than enough to hold a grown man under water. Caution anyone with long hair not to get near pool outlets. Long hair should be tied up or kept under a bathing cap.

Lifesaving. It is advisable that at least one person in every pool household have lifesaving and/or CPR training. When youngsters or nonswimmers will be using the pool, it's a good idea to install a safety line across the width of the pool, just before the point where the slope to the deep end begins. Mark the water depth clearly. Keep basic lifesaving equipment, such as a solid pole, a rope or a life ring, at poolside. If someone is in trouble and there is no proper safety equipment close by, throw something into the water that will float such as Styro-

foam toys or boards. Keep a complete first aid kit (the type available from the Red Cross) within easy reach, and post a list of emergency numbers at the phone nearest the pool. Keep the pool clean and clear of debris—you should be able to clearly see the bottom drain or bottom of the pool at all times.

Insurance. Once a pool has been installed, a home owner's insurance will be affected in two ways. A pool generally adds to the assessed value of the property, and it represents a significant liability as a home owner. In some states liability coverage is mandatory up to a particular amount. Your insurance agent will advise you as to the change of status and rate. Be sure you are properly covered from the very first day of pool operation.

Pool chemicals. Swimming pool chemicals are often in concentrated form and should be handled with thought and care. Carefully read and follow the instructions and warnings on the label of each product. Keep track of when chemicals were pur-

> Post a list of emergency numbers at the phone nearest the pool.

Do not allow swimming again until chemicals have dispersed for the specified amount of time.

chased; they may loose their effectiveness over time. Never mix various swimming pool chemicals together. Use a separate and clean scoop for each, and avoid combining "old" and "new" materials, even of the same product. Many chemicals, including different types of chlorine, can react violently when mixed, to produce toxic gases, fire, or explosion. Such chemicals are safe together only after they have been dissolved and dispersed in pool water. For this reason, pool chemicals should always be added to the pool water separately and according to the time specifications in the directions. Pour chemicals gently and try not to splash them. Keep the pool filter pump running to aid in rapid dispersion of the chemicals throughout the pool. Don't add chemicals to the pool while people are swimming; and do not allow swimming again until the chemicals have dispersed for the specified amount of time.

When stored, chemical containers must be tightly closed with their original lids. Store them in a clean, cool, dry, and well-ventilated area. Do not stack chemical containers.

Liquid and dry chemicals should be kept apart, and all other flammable items such as paints and fertilizers should also be kept out of the chemical storage area. Chemical fumes can corrode the metal of equipment and tools, so don't store pool chemicals near pumps, filters, or other metal mechanisms or tools. Chemicals of any kind should be stored well out of reach of curious children.

It bears repeating that when diluting pool chemicals before adding them to the pool, you always *add the chemicals to the water*. Never add water to dry or concentrated chemicals. When using chlorine, be careful not to inhale the fumes. If you use a chlorine tablet dispenser, do not add a different type of tablet to the one previously used, because there is the danger of severe reaction and even an explosion. Wash hands after handling chemicals. Remember that some chemicals are flammable—stay away from open flame or smoke when handling chemicals. If you decide to change the brand of chlorine tablet or stick, make sure the dispenser or basket is thoroughly rinsed to remove all residue of the former chemical.

15 • Hot Tubs and Spas

Hot tubs and spas have gained great popularity as vessels for relaxation and recreation in the home. Hot bathing is a practice that goes back to the ancient Romans, but didn't develop into a legitimate industry until the 1960s when wine and water vats were transformed into the earliest hot tub systems. Hot tubs and spas can be an alternative to a swimming pool if space or money are tight, they can enhance an outdoor swimming pool area, or can be brought under one's roof as part of a home addition or renovation project. Although they have elements similar to swimming pools, planning and caring for a wooden hot tub or fiberglass or Gunite spa is essentially different. The pages that follow will provide a brief introduction to the hot tub or spa as an alternative or addition to the swimming pool environment.

INSTALLATION CONSIDERATIONS

If you are installing a swimming pool, and think you might like to add a place for a hot soak, please keep in mind that it will be both easier to hook up, and more economical, to add one at the same time that the swimming pool is under construction. A tub or spa will certainly add a fair amount to the total cost of the installation, but it will cost you less in hassle and expense if you can combine the pool and tub/spa work.

There are a number of things to keep in mind when considering the addition of a hot tub or spa. Budget is, of course, something that must be established early. Decide on a preliminary dollar range within which you can reasonably afford to work. Hot tubs and spas can be as extravagant or austere as your imagination or plans permit. Some questions to ask early in the planning process include: what will it entail to prepare the site, what kind of materials do you think you would like to use, will it be enclosed or covered, will you want or need to do some landscaping, will you want much bubbling action, how many people do you want to accommodate? With answers in hand, do a little homework by contacting hot tub or spa contractors to see if you will fall above or below your preliminary budget. If you are not discouraged by the answers you get, then you can start to make some hard decisions.

Hot tubs and spas can be as extravagant or austere as your imagination or plans permit.

> Spas come in any conceivable size and shape. Most are made of molded fiberglass with a hard and smooth inner lining, but unlike tubs, they are not self-supporting.

A Hot Tub or Spa?

Your first choice is that between a hot tub or spa. This is often a personal decision, and not influenced as much by the conditions under which it will exist. In light of the descriptions that appear below, think about the setting you have planned (which would be more appropriate, hot tub or spa?), maintenance, and cost.

Hot tubs. These are self-supporting vessels made of hardwood, and are typically round- or oval-shaped with straight sides. A tub that is constantly filled with water will swell to perfect watertightness. Because it is extremely heavy when filled with water, the tub rests on concrete piers or blocks. The wood of choice among hot tub owners is vertical-grain, all-heart redwood. Noted for its attractive appearance, redwood is also resistant to decay. Other heartwoods used in hot tubs are cedar, cypress, oak, and even teak.

The average depth of a hot tub is 4 feet; the average diameter is be- tween 5 and 6 feet. Tubs in this range will hold approximately 600 gallons of water, and when you add three or four people the total weight can be 8,000 pounds. What hot tubs may have over spas is their portability because they are usually installed in above-grade locations. The most important drawback is that maintenance is crucial in a material such as wood. If you are vigilant, a hot tub can last more than a decade; without proper care, they can deteriorate over the course of a few years.

Spas. Your imagination and creativity can be more easily realized with spas because they come in any conceivable size and shape. Most are made of molded fiberglass with a hard and smooth inner lining, but unlike tubs, they are not self-supporting. You will need to prepare a spa site through excavation. The spa will be laid in the hole and then back-filled with sand. A reinforcing wall may be needed to hold up the sides against pressure from the water and bathers. Installation for spas will necessarily be more expensive be-

Photograph provided by the NSPI. Design: CSM Master Pools, Inc.; Belmont, California.

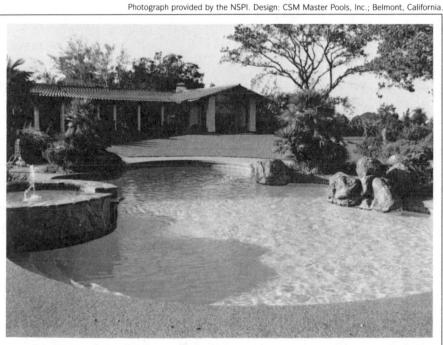

A pool and spa combination is hard to match for enjoyment, relaxation, and comfort.

A TYPICAL HOT TUB SET-UP

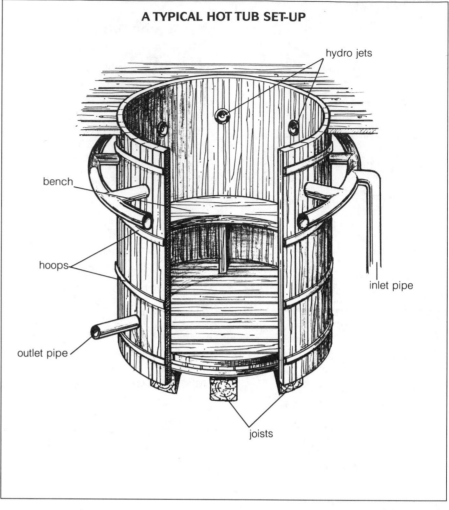

hydro jets

bench

hoops

outlet pipe

inlet pipe

joists

A TYPICAL SPA SET-UP

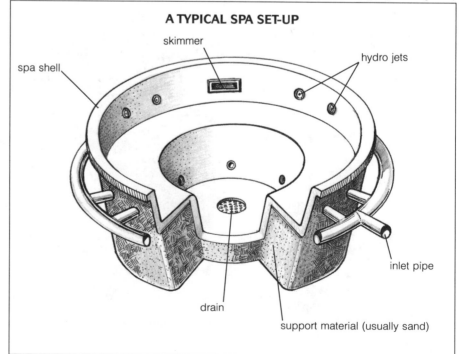

skimmer

spa shell

hydro jets

drain

inlet pipe

support material (usually sand)

WHAT COLOR IS YOUR SWIMMING POOL?

> The thing to consider in choosing a heater is *how much* you will be using the hot tub or spa, and *how fast* you want the water to reach the desired temperature.

cause the contractor will need to dig a hole, transport and deposit the spa shell to the site, and then backfill for support with sand. Spas are also made of concrete, masonry, Gunite, or metal, which is good to know in case a fiberglass shell is not right for your situation.

Spas are easier to keep clean and maintain because the surface is smooth and will not absorb chemicals and minerals in the way that hot tubs do. They are also shiny and attractive in a visual sense, and can be designed to fit any number of needs or desires. But once you have installed one, it is a permanent fixture. You need to be sure right from the start that a spa is what you really want.

The Support System and Accessories

The support system of any spa or hot tub is what separates them from a bath tub or vat of water. The components are much the same as those used in a swimming pool system, and some can even be shared with a swimming pool if you are installing the pool and tub or spa at the same time. The support system works as a unit to keep the circulating water clean and hot enough for a good soak, and accessories can add to your enjoyment and freedom from maintenance.

Pumps. The pump is really the heart of the system. Without it, water could not be pushed through the other components. The principle behind the pump is to suck the water in through an inlet, pump it through the filter, heater, bubblers, or jets, and then push it back into the hot tub or spa in a clean and warm condition. Your contractor or hot tub/spa professional will be the one to size the pump to the water capacity and circulating needs of the planned system.

Filters. The filter removes dirt and debris from the water by trapping it in, or behind, a medium such as

sand or a tightly-woven synthetic cartridge. There are three types of tub/spa filters to choose from: sand filter, diatomaceous (DE) filters, and cartridge filters. All are adequate for the needs of a hot tub or spa owner, and will remove even the most microscopic solids that can make the water cloudy or unhealthy, or which can inhibit the performance of other system components. Ask a contractor or professional which is best for the type of water in your area, and for the kind of use the hot tub or spa will probably get. Some filter systems are more expensive than others, so get prices for more than one kind of filter.

Heaters. The reason you are considering a hot tub or spa in the first place is to have hot, steaming water rushing around your body. The thing to consider in choosing a heater is *how much* you will be using the hot tub or spa, and *how fast* you want the water to reach the desired temperature. Different types of heaters can bring the water temperature up faster; others keep the water warm economically, but take longer to reach the hot soak range; and some will just cost you more to buy and keep operating at any rate. As with filters, investigate your options in light of anticipated usage and budget.

Jets and bubblers. Although most hot tubs or spas do include at least one of these features, they are really options. Do you want to have water swirling in from four sides or just two; do you want bubbles coming up all over? Hydro jets (or venturi jets) are really components that boost the force of the water coming into the hot tub or spa from the pump. These options will add to the cost and operating expense of the system, but they will also add to the enjoyment of the tub or spa.

Covers. A tub/spa cover will do a number of things for you. When the hot tub or spa is not in use, it will keep falling leaves, rain, trash, dirt,

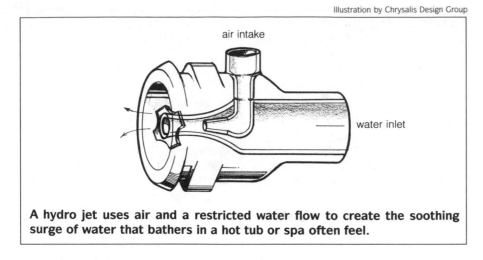

A hydro jet uses air and a restricted water flow to create the soothing surge of water that bathers in a hot tub or spa often feel.

and—most importantly—small children out of the water. Water that has been treated will suffer loss of its sanitizing chemicals if exposed to the sun and elements for any length of time. In addition, water temperature can be greatly diminished when allowed to sit without protection from wind, drafts, and ambient air conditions. As with pools, covers are an investment well worth making for hot tubs and spas.

Before you buy or build. Two things to remember as you embark on the hot tub or spa adventure. First, be a smart consumer: get prices or estimates from at least two manufacturers for each component, as well as from two contractors. Ask friends or neighbors about their hot tub/spa experience if you are comfortable with that. Second, secure all the appropriate building permits *before* work begins. Ask the contractor to show you building permits if you have hired someone else to do the work. In the event that you are tackling the job yourself, obtaining the permits in advance is your responsibility.

Finding a Home for Your Hot Tub or Spa

It may seem that there are infinite number of things to consider before a hot tub or spa can become a reality. It is the purpose of this book to help you make intelligent and thoughtful decisions. One of the most important decisions to make is exactly where the hot tub or spa will be located. But before you can know where the best place is, you have to understand your property and its landscape, the climate in your area, your relationship with your neighbors, and your family's life-style. If you have considered each of these things, you will make the right decision. Before you get too far, check into local zoning requirements (such as setback specifications) for tub/spa installations—this information can drastically alter your plans and the limit of possibilities.

Location. Make a rough map of your lot in which the house, trees, large plantings, and other features of the landscape or property (patios, steps, swing sets) are outlined. Walk around your lot and observe the following things: the grade of the land, how the sun falls at various times of the day, where the yard is exposed to wind or the neighbors' curious eyes, trees or shrubs that drop a disproportionate amount of debris (a tub/spa beneath a fruit tree would not be a good idea), where shadows fall, and where access to other underground utilities would be easiest. With these thoughts in your head, sketch two or three possible tub/spa

Before you get too far, check into local zoning requirements (such as setback specifications) for tub/spa installations—this information can drastically alter your plans and the limit of possibilities.

locations on your rough map. At least one of them should be right.

Weather. In some parts of the country you have to battle against the weather for a portion of the year, in others you can peacefully coexist with the elements all year long. There is no reason why the weather should hinder your decision to install a hot tub or spa, but it certainly can have a bearing on where you position it. Will you need protection from wind and the elements; will the sun and its seasonal shadows warm the water too much or transform it into an ice bath?

Indoor, outdoor, sheltered, framed? In light of the questions you have asked yourself from above, you may find that a shelter or framework of walls will be necessary. Or you may decide that despite your wish to have a tub outside your bedroom door, it will need to be completely enclosed. This is where an architect or designer can do the best job for you: they can come up with an imaginative and attractive plan that will fit your needs and your budget. Give that person your observations and wishes, and together you can come up with a mutually agreeable design.

Illustration by Chrysalis Design Group

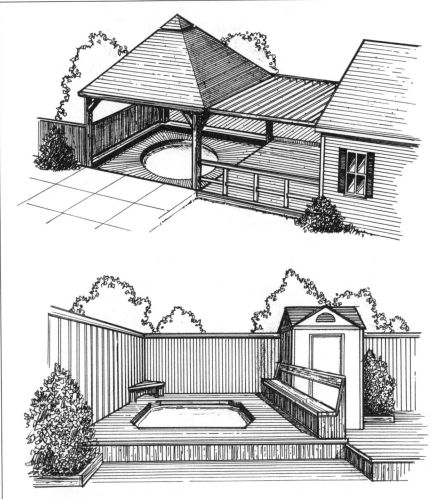

Hot tubs and spas will get greater use when they are designed to complement their surroundings and the lifestyle of their users. Benches, decking, enclosures, and fencing will all add to the appeal of a hot tub/spa installation.

WATER TREATMENT AND MECHANICAL MAINTENANCE

It is critical to keep tub or spa water well balanced. The ratio of people to the amount of circulating water is considerably smaller than a swimming pool; and higher temperatures break down the effectiveness of disinfectants, which encourages the growth of bacteria, algae, and mineral scale. When the water is clean and balanced, it is not only healthier for the bathers, but it is better for the proper operation of the mechanical components. A good place to start with water and equipment maintenance is to ask tub or spa bathers to shower with soap and water before entering. This regular practice will spare both the water and the equipment unnecessary treatment as a result of body grime, deodorants, and creams circulating through the system.

Taking Care of the Water

You will need four things to keep the tub/spa water in proper condition:

- A filter that operates 2 to 3 hours a day in good working order.
- A water quality test kit especially for the hot tub or spa (do not use the same kit to test pool water). It should include tests for pH, total alkalinity, chlorine or bromine, and water hardness.
- A disinfecting agent, either chlorine or bromine.
- Other water balancing or treatment chemicals: alkaline, acid, water clarifier, water softener, algaecide.

All these materials will be of no use unless you are disciplined about testing and balancing the water. The responsibility for clean water is not that of the filter or disinfectants—it is up to you.

pH. Water quality often begins and ends with pH. The recommended range for tub/spa water is between 7.2 and 7.6. Test for it every two or three days at the same time you test for disinfectant levels. If the pH has been allowed to rise or fall outside of this range, the water can quickly become cloudy, inhibit the effectiveness of chemicals, or corrode the support equipment. Soda ash will bring down the pH of water that is too alkaline; the addition of alkaline to the water will bring up the pH of water that is too acidic. Consult a tub/spa maintenance professional to get specific directions on how to attain the appropriate pH for your situation.

Aside from pH, total alkalinity and calcium hardness should be tested about every four weeks. The recommended range for total alkalinity is between 90 to 150 ppm; for hardness the range is more than 150 ppm, but less than 300 ppm. To learn how to correct readings outside of these parameters, you should consult a spa maintenance professional because it can be a complicated process. Once you understand how to correct and attain the right ppm reading for these two water balancing factors, you can do it yourself.

Disinfectants. Every spa or hot tub will need the addition of a chemical disinfectant to fight bacteria and algae growth. Disinfectants dissipate sooner in the hot water of tubs and spas, so more frequent water testing and treatment will be necessary. Chlorine and bromine are the disinfectants most widely used.

Assuming that every tub or spa owner will familiarize themselves with how to safely and effectively use chemical disinfectants, there are some things that bear emphasizing. Disinfectants should only be put into service by someone who has read the directions on the package carefully, and has a full knowledge of their properties. Do not run the

When the water is clean and balanced, it is not only healthier for the bathers, but it is better for the proper operation of the mechanical components. A good place to start with water and equipment maintenance is to ask tub or spa bathers to shower with soap and water before entering.

Liquid chlorine is not recommended for use in tubs or spas because it is too concentrated in this form for so small a body of water.

An annual inspection to look for, and remove, scale or mineral deposits on the heating elements when they become clearly visible is advised.

pump while the disinfectant is being added—it could hinder or damage the operation of the pump. Liquid chlorine is not recommended for use in tubs or spa because it is too concentrated in this form for so small a body of water. And last, be very careful to watch the clock and keep track of the time between the addition of more than one chemical to the tub or spa water—explosion or violent reaction could be the result of laziness or distraction.

Please follow these and other precautions for the safe handling of chemicals outlined by the NSPI in their materials on hot tubs and spas and on page 94 of this book.

Maintaining the Equipment

What follows hardly qualifies as thorough maintenance procedures for the tub/spa, pump, filter, and heater. This is because the maintenance procedure is pretty much the same for similar equipment in swimming pool systems. It's just the conditions under which tubs/spas and pools operate that is different. It is suggested that you obtain and read the maintenance manuals for each mechanical unit in your tub/spa system. Even if you call in a maintenance company or repair service, at least you will have a basic understanding of how to keep the tub/spa components operable.

Filters. It is advisable to clean or backwash the appropriate filter media once a month, or whenever the pressure gauge indicates that they need attention. Cartridges are removed and hosed off or scrubbed, then replaced; sand and DE filters are backwashed, and the filter medium replaced, if necessary.

Heaters. An annual inspection to look for, and remove, scale or mineral deposits on the heating elements when they become clearly visible is advised. Heater efficiency and its working life will be reduced when

such deposits are allowed to persist. Changing the tub/spa water regularly (every 2 or 3 months if possible in your area) should help avoid this condition.

Pumps and motors. These components are practically maintenance-free for the tub or spa owner. The most obvious regular chore is to remove the debris that gathers in the pump leaf strainer. The other thing you need to watch is that the pump does not lose its prime. If the prime fails, stop the motor immediately, fill it with water at the leaf strainer, securely replace the lid, and start the pump again. If this happens more than once within a short period of time, call in a tub/spa repairman.

It is extremely important to remember that before you work, clean, or tinker with any of the electrical equipment above that you turn off the power at the circuit breaker or fuse box. A good insurance practice is to have a licensed electrician inspect and test all equipment prior to its initial operation each swimming season, or once a year if the pool is in operation year-round.

HOT TUB AND SPA SAFETY

The owner of any recreational device —a boat, a pool, or a swing set—is responsible for seeing to it that the children or adults using it are well-supervised, follow established rules, and use good judgment. No less is true for the owners of hot tubs and spas. In many ways, a tub/spa owner must take greater care and caution because many people who are new to the hot tub experience may be at risk without even knowing it.

Water temperature. The single most important factor to remember is that the human body *cannot* withstand long soaks in water that is too hot. This practice is unsafe because it can raise the body's internal temperature, which can in turn raise the temperature of internal organs. Even a strong and healthy person can suffer organ failure in water that is deceivingly hot.

Keep an *accurate* thermometer in the hot tub or spa at all times, and check the temperature before and during use. Do not soak for more than 15 minutes at a time in water that is 104°F (40°C) or higher. If you prefer water at this temperature, leave the tub/spa after 15 minutes, shower, cool down, and return for another brief stay. The body can more reasonably tolerate long periods in water at a temperature of 98° or 99°F.

Around the tub or spa. A properly equipped tub or spa area should have a deck or steps with a slip-resis-tant surface that drains well to prevent puddles. Fences or doors with locks or self-closing latches can give you assurance against accidents or unwanted visitors. Handrails, steps, and ladders must be well-secured. If electrical outlets are part of the tub/spa design, have a licensed electrician do the work, and insist that ground fault interrupters (GFIs) be installed — they will protect against the hazards and disaster of electrical shock.

Chemicals. The best safety advice for the users of tub/spa chemicals is to follow the manufacturers' instructions for application and storage. Before you work with tub/spa chemicals, read the labels and corresponding directions carefully. Store all toxins, such as tub/spa chemicals, out of a child's reach.

> Do not soak for more than 15 minutes at a time in water that is 104°F (40°C) or higher.

Photograph provided by the NSPI. Design: Master Pools by Geremia Pools, Inc.; Sacramento, California.

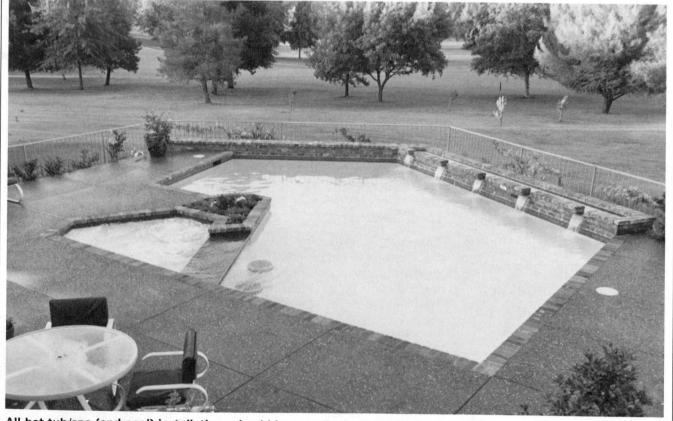

All hot tub/spa (and pool) installations should have a slip-resistant decking surface.

OTHER SAFETY TIPS

The following are safety tips that should be posted near the hot tub or spa. They are recommended and supplied by the NSPI, and should be observed by anyone using or supervising the tub/spa area.

- Pregnant women and persons suffering from heart disease, diabetes, or high or low blood pressure should not enter the spa/hot tub without prior medical consultation and permission from their doctor.
- Do not use the spa/hot tub while under the influence of alcohol, narcotics, or other drugs that cause sleepiness, drowsiness, or raise or lower blood pressure.
- Check spa/hot tub water temperature before use. Maximum safe temperature is 104°F (40°C).
- It is not advisable to use the hot tub or spa alone.
- Children should never use the tub or spa without adult supervision or when the water is very hot.
- Always enter and exit the tub/spa slowly.
- Observe reasonable time limits in the tub or spa to avoid nausea, dizziness, and fainting.
- Keep all breakable objects out of the tub/spa area.

- Electrical appliances should only be used near the tub or spa with the greatest of care. *Do not* use the telephone while soaking in the tub or spa — such a practice will invite disaster.
- Install ground fault interrupters to guard against electrical shock.
- Keep fingers, toes, and long hair away from grates and drains. The force of the pump can be enough to hold someone against them.
- Turn off the power before you begin any kind of work on the equipment and components.
- Emergency telephone numbers for police, fire, and rescue squad should be posted at the telephone nearest to the tub or spa.

It is highly recommended that all tub/spa owners obtain a copy of "The Sensible Way to Enjoy Your Spa or Hot Tub," which is available from the NSPI, and from which most of these safety tips derive. Every person that uses the tub/spa regularly should read it, and then as a group develop a list of rules for proper and safe use of the hot tub or spa.

Glossary

Acid. A chemical used to lower pH of pool water.

Acid demand. The amount of acid a pool requires to adjust the pH to the correct range.

Algae. Small plantlike organisms that grow in water. Algae discolors pool water and stains pool surfaces.

> Black algae. Algae that forms tough, dark-colored spots on pool surfaces—particularly visible in plaster pools.

> Green algae. Algae that grows in free-floating forms in the water and on pool walls; it is bright green in color.

> Mustard algae. A type of algae that grows on pool walls and is yellow, orange, or yellow-brown in color.

Algaecide. Chemical agent used to kill algae.

Alkalinity. A property of the water formed primarily by soluble salts—bicarbonates, carbonates, and hydroxides—which tends to increase pH.

Alum. A flocculating agent that causes dirt and other suspended particles in water to group together so they can more easily be removed by the filter. Potassium alum and ammonium alum are the most common types used.

Backwash. Reversing the flow direction of water in a filter to clean the filter of accumulated debris.

Bacteria. Minute unicellular organisms of various forms, some of which can cause disease.

Baking soda. Sodium bicarbonate that reacts with air and liquid to form carbon dioxide. It is one of many compounds of sodium elements, the most common of which is table salt (sodium chloride). In swimming pools, sodium bicarbonate (baking soda) is commonly used to raise the alkalinity of the water. It has the advantage over soda ash (sodium carbonate) in that baking soda does not raise the pH noticeably, whereas soda ash will raise pH.

Balanced water. Water that is neither corrosive nor scaling. Balanced water is achieved by proper adjustment of pH level, total alkalinity, calcium hardness, and total dissolved solids. These are the mineral constituents that water requires as its "food." If the water has less than the required minerals, the water is "hungry" or corrosive, obtaining minerals from metals in pool equipment and from plaster or concrete. When water has more minerals than it requires, the excess minerals are deposited onto pool surfaces and the interior of pipes and equipment as scale.

BROMINE. A chemical element used for water purification, particularly in hot tubs and spas. In a liquid state it is a dark, heavy, reddish-brown liquid, but it is most often sold in stick or tablet form.

CALCIUM CARBONATE. The combination of carbonate ions and calcium ions. In balanced water, calcium remains in the water as calcium ions. High pH and/or total alkalinity increase the number of carbonate ions that can combine with calcium ions to produce visible calcium carbonate precipitation.

CALCIUM HARDNESS. A term to indicate the mineral content of water. Water obtains these minerals, primarily calcium and magnesium, from rocks and other solids over which water moves. The average hardness of surface waters in the U.S. varies from under 60 ppm in the Northwest, Southeast, and Northeast to over 240 ppm in some central states. Hardness is a disadvantage for household applications, but in pool water hardness helps to protect pool surfaces from the corrosive effects of water. *See also* HARDNESS.

CALCIUM HYPOCHLORITE. A dry form of chlorine (usually 65 percent average chlorine by weight) in combination with calcium.

CARTRIDGE FILTER. A pool water filter may contain paper or polyester cartridges as the filter medium.

CHEMICAL FEEDER. A device used to feed (and sometimes meter) chemicals into the pool. Types include injection feeders, proportioning pumps, pot feeders, and dry feeders.

CHLORAMINES. Chemical compounds formed when chlorine comes in contact with ammonia (from garden fertilizers, urine, or body sweat and oils). Chloramines are not effective as sanitizers and produce burning eyes and skin irritation. They are usually responsible for the chlorine odor in pool water. Contrary to popular belief, eye irritation and a strong chlorine smell do not indicate that there is too much chlorine in the water, but that there is *too little chlorine*.

CHLORINATION. The addition of chemicals containing chlorine to sanitize pool water.

CHLORINATOR. A device that dispenses, regulates, and meters the amount of chlorine introduced into water on a semiautomatic or fully automatic basis.

CHLORINE. An oxidizing chemical sanitizer widely used in water purification and pool water sanitizing. Chlorine kills algae and bacteria, and oxidizes (burns up) suspended dirt particles in water. It is available in a liquefied gas form, stored under pressure in cylinders for PROFESSIONAL APPLICATION ONLY. For use by pool owners, chlorine comes in much safer forms—liquid, powder, tablet, or stick.

CHLORINE DEMAND. The quantity of chlorine required to destroy pollutants in the pool (bacteria, algae, chloramines). Once this "demand" is satisfied, a small residual amount of "free chlorine" becomes available in the water to keep it in a sanitary condition.

CHLORINE RESIDUAL. The amount of chlorine available for sanitizing after the initial chlorine demand of the water has been met. Also known as free chlorine or free available chlorine. Chlorine residual should be maintained at 1.0 to 1.5 ppm in a stabilized pool.

CYANURIC ACID. A mild acid of low toxicity with little effect on pH. It is added to pool water to retard the loss of chlorine due to sunlight. *Chlorinated isocyanurics* are chlorine mixtures that contain cyanuric acid. Such chlorine mixtures, called *stabilized chlorine*, include calcium hypochlorite and trihydroxy triazine.

DIATOMACEOUS EARTH (DE). A fine, powderlike substance consisting of the compressed, powdered skeletons of tiny prehistoric diatoms. DE is used as a filter media (septum) for swimming pools, in breweries and in the recovery of solvents used in dry-cleaning establishments.

DISCHARGE HEAD. The total head (pressure of fluid) on the discharge side of a water pump.

DISTRIBUTOR. The device used in a pool filter to divert incoming water and prevent erosion of the filter media (for example, the sand in a sand filter).

ELECTROLYSIS. An electron flow (migration of ions) between two dissimilar metals submerged in water, which causes corrosion.

FREE CHLORINE. *See* CHLORINE RESIDUAL.

FILTER CYCLE. The length of operating time between backwash cycles of the filter, or how long the filter will operate before it needs to be backwashed (cleaned).

FILTER RATE. The rate of water flow through a filter, expressed in gallons per minute per square foot of filter area. Usually stamped on the manufacturer's plate on the filter housing.

FLOCCULATING AGENT. A compound, such as alum, that causes small particles of suspended dirt or other materials to clump together into larger masses. *See also* ALUM.

FLOW RATE. Volume of flow per unit of time expressed in gallons per minute (GPM).

GUNITE. A trademark name for the process of spraying a concrete mixture under pressure over steel reinforcing rods. The term Gunite is often used in place of pneumatically applied concrete, which is the technical term. Gunite application is called a "dry" process, in that the concrete mixture is not premixed before application—water is added to the mixture in the nozzle of the Gunite gun as it is being applied.

HARDNESS. The amount of calcium and magnesium dissolved in water. High levels of these minerals in *unbalanced* water can cause scale and cloudy water. Low levels cause water to "attack" and corrode pool surfaces and equipment. High levels of calcium and magnesium in *balanced* water contribute to protection of plaster and metals.

HYPOCHLORINATOR. A device used to dispense chlorine to a pool. It contains a mixing tank and feeds a controlled amount of chlorine to the pool.

HYPOCHLORITE. Any salt form of hypochlorous acid (chlorine).

CALCIUM HYPOCHLORITE. A powder or tablet form of chlorine that contains about 70 percent pure chlorine.

SODIUM HYPOCHLORITE. This is the most common liquid form of chlorine for pool sanitizing. It contains about 16 percent chlorine (household bleach has about 5 percent chlorine). It disperses quickly in water, doesn't add to water hardness, but does raise pH and alkalinity.

HYPOCHLOROUS ACID. The most active sanitizing agent in chlorine. Formed when chlorine is added to water, hypochlorous acid production is controlled by the pH level of the water.

INFLUENT. Water entering the pool through a filter or other device.

INLET. A fitting or port through which water passes to the pool.

MAIN OUTLET/DRAIN. The outlet or drain in the bottom of the deepest part of the pool, through which water is drawn to the circulating pump and filter.

MULTIPORT VALVE. A valve having at least four control positions for various filter operations.

MURIATIC ACID. A commercial form of hydrochloric acid, used to lower the pH of pool water and for etching and acid-washing pool surfaces.

OTO (ORTHOTOLIDINE). A solution (reagent) used in a pool water test kit to measure the amount of residual or free chlorine present.

OUTLET LINE. A pipe or pipes from the main drain and/or skimmers used to pump water from the pool to the pump and filter.

OVERFLOW GUTTER. A gutter around the top of some pools, used to carry away waste from the surface water to the filter and to catch the water displaced by swimmers.

OXIDATION. The action or union of oxygen with another substance. In pool water, hypochlorous acid (chlorine) oxidates (burns up) algae, bacteria, and suspended dirt particles.

pH. Potential hydrogen. A scale of numbers from 1 to 14 used to indicate the acidity or alkalinity of pool water. A neutral solution is represented by a measure of 7. Readings below 7 indicate an acidic condition; readings above 7 indicate an alkaline condition. Desired pH range for pool water is 7.2 to 7.6.

PPM. Parts per million. For example, 2 ppm salt means that in 1 million pounds of water or other solution, there are 2 pounds of salt.

PRESSURE DIFFERENTIAL. The difference in pressure between two or more actions of a hydraulic system, such as the difference in pressure between the inlet flow and outlet flow of a pump or filter.

RECIRCULATING SYSTEM. The complete water filtration system, consisting of pipes, pump, strainer, filter, and skimmer.

RESIDUAL CHLORINE. See CHLORINE RESIDUAL.

RETURN LINE. The pipe (or outlet line) that connects the filter outlet to the pool. Automatic chlorinators and chemical dispensers are plumbed into this line.

SHOCK TREATMENT. The addition of pool chemicals in larger-than-normal amounts in order to eliminate unusual pool water conditions such as infestations of algae, the presence of chloramines or colored water. See also SUPERCHLORINATION.

SHOTCRETE. Another trademark name for spraying concrete under pressure, but unlike Gunite, Shotcrete uses a "wet" concrete mixture already premixed. With Shotcrete it is important that the time between premixing and application not be long, to avoid the problem of concrete curing prior to application, which can later cause cracks in the concrete.

SKIMMER. A device to remove leaves and other floating debris from the water surface. A *manual skimmer* is a flat net on the end of a long pole. An *automatic skimmer* is usually built into the side of the pool, connected by pipes to the pump/filter unit.

SLURRY. A watery mixture (not a solution) of diatomaceous earth or chlorine powder, or a mixture of water and cement or plaster.

SODA ASH. Common name for sodium carbonate, a dry chemical used to increase the pH (alkalinity) of pool water.

SODIUM BICARBONATE. See BAKING SODA.

SODIUM BISULFATE. A compound of sodium and acid sulfate (also called sodium and acid sulfate or dry acid) that can be used to bring the pH down in water through an increase of hydrogen ions.

SODIUM HYPOCHLORITE. *See* HYPOCHLORITE.

STABILIZATION. The addition of a stabilizer or conditioner, such as cyanuric acid, to pool water to extend the effective life of chlorine by protecting it from the dissipating effects of sunlight.

SUPERCHLORINATION. Addition of larger-than-normal amounts of chlorine during periods of excessive heat or rainfall and heavy pool use, to convert chloramines into free available chlorine by destroying ammonia.

TOTAL ALKALINITY (TA). The measurement of all alkaline chemicals in the pool water. A total alkalinity (TA) that is too high causes the pH to resist adjustment to the desired range. When the TA is too low, it is difficult to maintain the pH within the desired range.

TURNOVER RATE. The time it takes for a pool's circulation system to pass a volume of water through the filter equal to the amount of water contained in the pool. Usually expressed in hours.

VACUUM WALL FITTING. A fitting in the pool wall below the waterline for attaching the hose of a pool vacuum (suction) hose. In some pools, the vacuum fitting is located in the skimmer box.

WEIR. Originally a low dam or obstruction placed in a stream. In swimming pool usage, it refers to the small hinged plate in the "throat" or inlet of a skimmer box. It is this weir flap that gives the skimming action. The weir contains a buoyant section so that it floats high in the water, allowing only about three-sixteenths of an inch of surface water to flow into the skimmer box.

Index